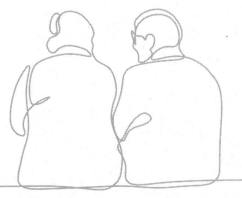

Neglected No More

The Urgent Need to
Improve the Lives of Canada's Elders
in the Wake of a Pandemic

ANDRÉ PICARD

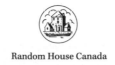

Random House Canada

PUBLISHED BY RANDOM HOUSE CANADA

Copyright © 2021 André Picard

www.penguinrandomhouse.ca

Random House Canada and colophon are registered trademarks.

Library and Archives Canada Cataloguing in Publication

Title: Neglected no more : the urgent need to improve the lives of
Canada's elders in the wake of a pandemic /André Picard.
Names: Picard, André, 1960– author.
Identifiers: Canadiana (print) 20200281488 | Canadiana (ebook) 20200281496
ISBN 9780735282247 (softcover) | ISBN 9780735282254 (EPUB)
Subjects: LCSH: Older people—Care—Canada. | LCSH: Long-term care facilities—
Canada. | LCSH: Older people—Home care—Canada.
Classification: LCC HV1475.A3 P53 2021 | DDC 362.60971—dc23

Text design: Matthew Flute
Cover design: Matthew Flute
Image credits: (elderly couple) © Tetiana Garkusha / iStock / Getty

Printed and bound in Canada

2 4 6 8 9 7 5 3 1

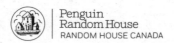

Penguin
Random House
RANDOM HOUSE CANADA

CONTENTS

Introduction

When eldercare makes headlines in Canada, it's usually news of the worst kind.

On June 26, 2017, former nurse Elizabeth Wettlaufer was sentenced to life in prison for murdering eight vulnerable elders in care homes where she worked in southwestern Ontario. The inquiry that followed concluded that, had she not confessed, Wettlaufer would never have been caught.

Just after midnight on January 23, 2014, a blaze broke out in the kitchen of the Résidence du Havre nursing home in L'Isle-Verte, Quebec. Thanks to a lack of sprinklers, the absence of staff to help frail residents escape and the inept emergency response that followed, thirty-two residents suffered horrific deaths. No one was ever charged.

On January 20, 2019, 93-year-old Hélène Rowley Hotte, the mother of former Bloc Québécois leader Gilles Duceppe, left her seniors' residence in response to a (false) fire alarm, without anyone on staff noticing. The emergency exit door locked behind her. That night the temperature in Montreal dipped to minus-21 degrees Celsius, and Hélène Rowley Hotte froze to death. A coroner's inquest ruled the death was preventable but accidental. No one was charged.

Then came Covid-19.

As the novel coronavirus slithered into unprepared long-term-care homes, elders were no longer dying one at a time, or even by the dozens, but by the hundreds and thousands. Those deaths too were largely preventable. You can bet your lunch that no individual or organization will be held to account for the mass death of vulnerable seniors.

Eldercare in this country is so disorganized and so poorly regulated, the staffing so inadequate, the infrastructure so outdated, the accountability so non-existent and ageism so rampant, there seems to be no limit to what care homes can get away with.

Of course, there will be the obligatory inquiry. When a gross societal failure occurs, you can always count on Canadian politicians to embrace obfuscation and foot-dragging in lieu of action. In her 1,491-page report, Madam Justice Eileen Gillese, the Ontario Court of Appeal judge who presided over the Public Inquiry into the Safety and Security of Residents in the Long-Term Care Homes System (the Wettlaufer inquiry), said the reason a killer can run amok, undetected, is "systemic vulnerabilities." She concluded that "assigning blame to individuals or organizations is counterproductive."

That's pretty much the conclusion of every coroner's report, judicial inquiry and investigation that has ever been conducted into failings such as those cited above. And, remember, those cases are just the tip of the iceberg, the spectacular failures that generate media attention and political hand-wringing, not the everyday neglect that is deadly too. Yet the "systemic vulnerabilities" that are exposed time and time again never seem to get corrected. In Canadian health care, it seems, no screw-up, no matter how big or small, how sickening or deadly, is ever anyone's fault. It's always the fault of "the system."

So let's fix the damn system.

Neglected No More isn't a book about Covid-19, except periph-erally. It's a plea to stop dehumanizing elders, and to reimagine long-term care (LTC). It tells of families frustrated by their inability to access the care their loved ones want, the angst of dedicated workers who don't have the time or resources to deliver the care elders want and need, and how a combination of history, changing demographics, political inertia and a health system with other pri-orities created a proverbial perfect storm that allowed a pathogen to ravage a vulnerable population.

It's not a call for heads to roll that will never roll. It's a stark exposé of what's wrong and a rough blueprint for what we need to do to fix eldercare.

When I first wrote about AIDS in 1981, the acronym had yet to be coined; the strange new illness, which seemed to affect only gay men, was dubbed GRID—gay-related immune deficiency. In the four decades since, AIDS has become, arguably, the most deadly pandemic in human history. At least 36 million people have died of AIDS, and another 40 million are still living with HIV, the human immunodeficiency virus that causes AIDS. (Of course, nothing compares to the Black Death. The bubonic plague killed some-where between 75 and 200 million people between 1346 and 1353. But that was long before the advent of medicine or public health measures such as sanitation and clean water.)

AIDS has not only described the arc of my career in journalism, it has spawned in me a long-standing interest in pathogens more broadly: the viruses, bacteria, fungi, parasites, worms and prions that have been the scourge of humanity since the dawn of time. I have written about all manner of infectious micro-organisms, from the obscurely rare to those that casually kill millions a year, everything from sleeping sickness to tuberculosis, chicken pox to Ebola, polio to influenza.

Outbreaks rarely generate much media attention. The exception was Severe Acute Respiratory Syndrome (SARS). In 2003, SARS-CoV killed forty-four Canadians, devastated the economy and exposed gaping holes in our public health infrastructure. It was a dress rehearsal for a real pandemic.

The formal name for the pandemic virus that causes Covid-19 is SARS-CoV-2. When it arrived in our midst, someone (I wish I could remember who) said, "You've been training for this moment your whole life." That's true. For me, infectious diseases are fascinating not because of their biology, but because they almost always have wide-ranging social, economic and political implications.

We are only beginning to get a sense of the earth-shattering fallout from Covid-19. In Canada, the pandemic has, among other things, exposed the fault lines in our institutions—political, public health, judicial and more. But no sector has been more brutally unmasked than eldercare, the hodgepodge of long-term-care homes, home care and affordable housing for seniors that lurks on the margins of health and welfare systems. We have long deluded ourselves into thinking our elders were well cared for. Now the norm has been shown to be horribly inadequate. We have been forced to confront the fact that the old way of doing things—dispatching our elders to live in holding-on-by-a-shoestring nursing homes—is not working.

AIDS forced journalists to write about all manner of issues that were largely taboo until then: homophobia, intravenous drug use, sex work, institutionalized misogyny and more. It made us confront uncomfortable socio-economic realities such as how poverty, marginalization and disempowerment are pathogens' best friends. Covid-19 is reminding us that we need to relearn many of those lessons.

It is hard to imagine a population that has been more profoundly neglected for an extended period than elders. The responses to the sickening incidents cited at the outset of this introduction exposed multiple "systemic vulnerabilities"—the treatment of elders as disposable, understaffing, poor regulation and a total absence of accountability—that were never corrected. If anything, they grew worse. That set the stage for what happened in care facilities during Covid-19: thousands upon thousands of deaths, most of which were preventable.

What is perhaps most shocking is how little was done to raise the ramparts around nursing homes. Anyone with even a passing knowledge of infectious diseases would know that frail seniors living in congregate settings are sitting ducks for pathogens, especially respiratory viruses. As soon as the word "pandemic" was uttered, alarm bells should have gone off and protective measures put in place.

That elders were at high risk was no secret. By February 2020, there was extensive coverage describing how coronavirus was hitting seniors particularly hard in China and in Europe, and warning that this phenomenon could soon hit North America. Among people over the age of 80 who had contracted coronavirus, the death rate was 22 percent; in those aged 70 to 80, it was 8 percent.

The headline on a column I wrote in the March 8 edition of the *Globe and Mail*—before a single nursing home death had occurred—read: SENIOR CARE FACILITIES ARE ESPECIALLY VULNERABLE TO COVID-19 OUTBREAKS. Not long after that, I wrote another column saying "if you can get your relatives out of seniors' homes, try to do it as fast as you can." That commentary triggered many angry responses, but, in retrospect, my only regret is not having said it sooner.

It would take almost two months before politicians officially acknowledged the severity of the long-term-care crisis, by calling in the troops, literally. Canadian Forces health specialists were deployed to the hardest-hit homes in late April 2020. By then, thousands had already died. Quebec, the hardest-hit province by far, created "SWAT teams" to dispatch to care homes in October 2020, but did so only after a second round of deaths in institutional care was well under way.

The way elders died—almost always alone, their family caregivers locked out, without palliative care, and often with little care at all—was the greatest horror of all. Nihilism reared its head in our public policy response, an underlying ageist "they're going to die anyhow" attitude. The proponents of "herd immunity"—let the coronavirus run rampant and if vulnerable elders die en masse, too bad, that's the price of getting the economy running at full steam—openly reflected this crude philosophy.

There are those who will be looking for villains—politicians, care home operators, workers who walked off the job. But the real villain in this tragedy is society's profound and long-standing neglect of elders. A reckoning is in order.

Part One

NEGLECTED

CHAPTER 1

The Covid-19 Horror Show

On the evening of March 29, 2020, a small group of local public health officials walked into Résidence Herron, a 134-bed private long-term-care facility in the Montreal suburb of Dorval. They didn't know exactly what to expect, but the scene they confronted was stomach-churning: Residents wallowing in their own urine and feces because their incontinence pads had not been changed in days. Others sitting in wheelchairs and lying on soiled bedsheets, dehydrated, hungry and disoriented, having not been fed or given their medications. Two patients on the verge of death. Two overwhelmed orderlies and one other employee were the only staff left on site, instead of the fifteen who would normally be working the day shift. The rest had quit or simply disappeared, and management was nowhere to be found either.

The first action the officials took was to call in a cadre of nurses to deliver emergency personal care: feeding, bathing and dressing residents. Upon reviewing patient files, the nurses discovered that a number of residents had died of Covid-19 at the care facility in the previous two weeks, but little had been done to protect those who remained, dozens of whom were believed to be infected.

The outbreak at Herron was not the first in a Canadian long-term-care facility, nor would it be the last. It was far from the worst, at least in terms of fatalities. But the story, which would only come to light publicly almost two weeks later, graphically underscored just how chaotic and dire the situation had become in a great many eldercare facilities, and just how disruptive and deadly coronavirus would prove to be for those living in institutional care.

It was less than three weeks after the World Health Organization had declared Covid-19 a global pandemic, and Canadians were just waking up to how devastating it could be. As the pandemic swept around the world, it shone a spotlight on many existing social woes, not the least of which was how our elders have been neglected and forgotten. The crisis also exposed a tragic reality: the generation that had given Canada its beloved medicare system had clearly been forsaken by it.

On December 31, 2019, Helen Branswell, a Canadian journalist working for Stat News, posted a link on Twitter about reports of "unexplained pneumonias" in the Hubei province in China. The tweet referenced chatter on ProMed, an e-mail list and website that serves as an early warning system for infectious diseases, and which is a favourite of a geeky subset of scientists, physicians and reporters. Ms. Branswell said the news was giving her "SARS flashbacks," a quip that would prove incredibly prescient. Later that day, the Wuhan Municipal Health Commission would issue a brief report officially acknowledging the outbreak, which media reports said had originated at a seafood market in Wuhan, a port city of 11 million people.

On January 7, 2020, Chinese officials said the respiratory illness was caused by a novel coronavirus, which would later be named SARS-CoV-2. The virus originated in bats (which are known to harbour many coronaviruses) and was probably transmitted to humans via an animal host, likely pangolins, one of the many exotic animals sold at the market. By January 12, China had already decoded the genome of the virus and published it. At the time, there had been only forty-one identified cases and one death. In global public health circles, alarm bells were starting to go off, but the belief was that the virus could be contained to China, which had already begun to impose what would become the largest quarantine in history.

Canada recorded its first case on January 25, a Toronto man in his 50s who had just returned from Wuhan. He was placed in isolation at Sunnybrook Hospital. At a hastily arranged press conference, six dour Ontario health officials said they were monitoring the situation closely but there was no need to worry because Canada was better prepared this time.

The implied "last time" was March 7, 2003, a day when two men with serious respiratory symptoms walked into two different Canadian hospitals—one in Toronto and the other in Vancouver. SARS, caused by a novel coronavirus that likely spread from civets sold in Chinese markets, would eventually kill 774 people and sicken 8,098 in thirty-seven countries before it disappeared.

The hardest-hit country outside Asia was Canada, which recorded forty-four deaths and 3,301 hospitalizations, almost all of them in the province of Ontario. SARS, which spread almost exclusively in hospitals because of poor infection control measures, also caused billions of dollars in economic losses as visitors avoided Toronto.

The SARS crisis prompted a lot of introspection in Canada, including two public inquiries that gave us the 1,200-page opus *Spring of Fear* from the SARS Commission, led by Mr. Justice Archie Campbell, and the more modest 234-page tome *Learning from SARS*, by the National Advisory Committee on SARS, headed by Dr. David Naylor. The take-home message of these two in-depth analyses could be boiled down to the Boy Scout motto "Be prepared"—because there was no doubt other infectious disease threats were on the horizon, and the response had to be more swift and nimble than it had been with SARS.

In response, the federal government created the Public Health Agency of Canada and the hardest-hit province formed a body called Public Health Ontario. British Columbia, the only other province affected by SARS, bolstered its public health infrastructure too. Significant money was spent to create stockpiles of emergency equipment such as masks, respirators and ventilators. Hospitals built negative pressure rooms to minimize the risk that pathogens could spread within the institution. Committees were formed. Minutely detailed pandemic preparedness plans were also drafted, which included everything from "social distancing" (a term that would soon enter Canadians' everyday lexicon) to "management of mass fatalities." When the next pandemic threat came along, Canada vowed that it was going to be supremely prepared. And it was, sort of.

When it became clear that the novel coronavirus was spreading outside China, all the attention was on travellers, on ensuring that anyone who carried the virus in from another country would be identified and isolated quickly. During SARS, the early cases among travellers were detected only after they were hospitalized and had already infected other patients and staff. This time around, hospitals would be ready. They began implementing their pandemic plans, which included freeing up as many beds as possible in preparation for a possible surge in patients.

One of the reasons hospitals in Canada are chronically overcrowded is that many patients are classified as needing an "alternate level of care"—which means they have care needs that can't be provided in their homes and yet there is no room in care facilities where they want to be placed. As the Covid-19 pandemic took hold, many of these patients were dispatched to nursing homes and long-term-care homes anyway, ostensibly for their own safety. After all, based on the heartbreaking scenes in hospitals in Italy and Spain, Canada could soon be facing a crisis of its own, and no one wanted a repeat of SARS, or worse. Hospitals had to be protected—at all costs.

On March 26, Herron reported its first official case of Covid-19, a patient who was transferred to the Jewish General Hospital, where she died. The next day, several more residents were sent to hospital. Many staff members were told to quarantine as a precautionary measure, and the facility struggled to find replacements for them. There is much debate, some of it taking place in legal proceedings, about how much effort owners of the home made to replace staff. What is not in doubt is that, as the virus spread, residents were not getting the basic personal care they needed for several days. On March 29, a physician visiting Herron called 911 because her patient was quite ill. When paramedics arrived, they found only three workers on site to care for 133 residents, and one of the workers was quite ill. They notified local public health authorities.

The director of the local public health authority, Lynne McVey, decided to go see for herself, and she brought reinforcements. The scene that greeted them was "akin to a concentration camp," according to an anonymous source cited in a *Montreal Gazette* story that exposed the scandal. Loredana Mule, a veteran registered nurse (RN) who volunteered to help with what essentially became a rescue mission, was stunned by the sight of dozens of frightened, emaciated seniors. "I'd never seen anything like it in my 32-year nursing career," she said. "It was horrific—there wasn't enough food to feed people, the stench could've killed a horse." She and three other nurses worked for sixteen hours straight to get residents fed, bathed and dressed. "When we finished, I went to my car and cried," she said. Then, the next day, she pulled her own mother out of the seniors' residence where she lived, convinced that she would be safer at home.

It would be revealed later that there had been Covid-19 cases in Herron weeks earlier, around the time a provincial lockdown of care homes took effect on March 14. At that point, coronavirus was spreading rapidly, so care homes were supposed to have a separate "red zone" for infected people and a "yellow zone" for those awaiting test results. But there is little evidence the sick at Herron were isolated, or that staff took any special precautions with their care, such as wearing personal protective equipment (PPE). It was business as usual until everything fell apart spectacularly.

Peter Wheeland, a freelance writer and translator, had both his parents living at Herron. Their journey from independent living to institutional care is one familiar to many Canadian families.

Ken and Connie Wheeland lived in the same bungalow in the Montreal borough of Dollard-des-Ormeaux for almost six decades, raising five children. In 2015, then aged 81 and 82 respectively, with health woes making it increasingly difficult to navigate and maintain the home, they decided to move to a seniors' residence. But over a couple of years, Mrs. Wheeland developed mobility problems due to severe arthritis in her knees. When the complex staged a fire drill and she was unable to leave the building on her own, she was deemed too high-risk to live there.

Her husband, who was still in good health, went looking for an alternative, a facility where they could still live as a couple and get the care his wife needed, and which he might need in the coming years. He settled on Résidence Herron, a private, for-profit home. "In hindsight, I wish they had looked at other options," says their son Peter. "These are difficult decisions and no one helps seniors make the right choices."

In the fall of 2019, Ken Wheeland began to experience frequent falls, along with memory problems. He was diagnosed with vascular dementia and his health deteriorated quickly. He was in and out of hospital regularly and, back at Herron, he spent most of his time in bed, and developed severe pressure ulcers (also known as bedsores). "To me that was a clear sign they weren't taking good care of him," Peter Wheeland says.

People who are bed-bound need to be rotated at least every two hours to ensure they don't develop painful and life-threatening pressure ulcers, since infections of the sores are a common cause of death. When Peter complained, administrators said that his father was not paying for the level of care required, and they would need to raise the cost for him to live at Herron to $5,000 monthly, from the $3,200 he was already paying. (Connie Wheeland was being charged $4,000 monthly.) For the family, the price hike was the last straw, not to mention unaffordable, and they arranged to move their father to a publicly funded long-term-care home. They hoped their mother would soon be able to join him there.

Then Covid-19 hit. Quebec, like every other province, attempted to vacate hospital beds to prepare for a surge of patients afflicted with the virus. But at the same time, the province continued to admit seniors to long-term care, even after reports of hundreds of outbreaks. The first Covid-19 case in the province, a traveller who had just returned from Iran, was on February 28, and the first case in a seniors' facility was March 12. Yet even as case numbers were rising exponentially, new admissions to long-term-care facilities continued until April 10, the day the *Montreal Gazette* exposé on the horrors at Herron was published.

On March 17, Ken Wheeland left the private Résidence Herron in a taxi, and was dropped off at the public CHSLD LaSalle. (In Quebec, long-term-care homes are known by the initialism CHSLD, which stands for Centre d'hébergement de soins de longue durée.) Soon after he arrived at the CHSLD, Ken developed breathing problems. "We didn't know if he had Covid, but we suspected," Peter recalls. A few days later, a media report revealed that there was a large outbreak at the home. Family members could not visit Ken and couldn't speak to him by phone either, since the technicians who installed phones were no longer allowed in the building. Eventually, the family managed to get Ken a cellphone, but he grew so ill that calls were few and far between.

On April 4, at age 85, Ken Wheeland died. Family members had been allowed a brief visit to say goodbye; his wife of sixty-three years had only a short phone call. The next day, it was confirmed that he had died of Covid-19. It is not clear whether he was infected at Herron or at LaSalle, but the way he was shuffled around without being tested, and while facilities were supposed to be locked down, helps illustrate how coronavirus was spreading like wildfire through care facilities.

Meanwhile, the family had little idea what was going on at Herron. When Peter Wheeland learned that the local public health unit had come into the home with extra staff, he was actually relieved. "I felt like the cavalry had finally arrived." His mother was getting fed and changed, and she had her first bath in weeks. Like the whole family, she was grieving Ken, but no funerals were allowed during the pandemic. The family was also concerned that Connie might be infected with Covid-19, although they were comforted by media reports that Herron had only three cases and they were all being treated in hospital. But it turned out the home's co-owner, Samir Chowieri, had left out quite a few details, notably about chronic staffing problems that grew markedly worse during the pandemic.

On April 10, the blockbuster *Montreal Gazette* story revealed, among other things, that during a two-week period, from March 13 to 29, thirty-one people in the home had died of Covid-19 before public health authorities were even informed. Ill-equipped to handle the outbreak, and fearing for their own health and that of their families, many workers simply stopped showing up, leaving surviving residents in dire straits. (This problem was not unique to Herron. At his daily press briefing, Premier François Legault begged "missing" health workers to return to the job; there were as many as 9,500 a day who failed to do so at the peak of the out break.) The death toll at Herron would eventually rise to sixty-one, a 44 percent mortality rate. Normally, the home recorded only two to four deaths monthly.

Danielle McCann, Quebec's Minister of Health and Social Services, ordered that the home be placed under trusteeship and that the ministry conduct an inquiry. At a press conference the day the *Gazette* story was published, Premier Legault seemed visibly angry. He called the situation at the home "deplorable" and "unacceptable," and said "it certainly seems like gross negligence." Mr. Legault added that he had asked police to investigate whether criminal charges were warranted against Herron's owners.

The owners, Groupe Katasa, tried to deflect blame onto public authorities, saying they had created chaos when they stepped in, allowing infected and non-infected patients to mingle. The problem with that explanation was that patients had been dying for weeks before the intervention, and no one was tested unless they were transferred to hospital.

Herron was built in 1988, making it a relatively new facility; many care homes in the province were built decades, and sometimes more than a century, ago. It also wasn't cheap, charging clients as much as $10,000 monthly. Still, it had been cited for poor care by inspectors in the past. In 2017 the Protecteur du citoyen, the provincial ombudsperson, did a more in-depth investigation in response to numerous complaints from families. The report cited a long list of deficiencies, including inadequate staffing, poorly trained staff, a shortage of essential supplies such as incontinence pads, a lack of variety in the food service, an ineffective complaints procedure, and poor communication with families, especially about financial aspects. In 2019, the provincial coroner also issued a damning report about the quality of care at Herron after a 94-year-old resident choked to death on her food.

The mass deaths at Herron triggered a flurry of legal responses. In addition to the police investigation and the Ministry of Health review, there was a coroner's inquest specific to Herron, and another looking at the response to Covid-19 in homes across the province, and there will likely be a broad public inquiry as well. The first of the reports that was issued, in September 2020, said the root of the disaster was "organizational negligence"—in other words, the owners had no idea how to run a care home. Several families of those who died at Herron also filed a class action lawsuit, alleging "inhuman and degrading maltreatment" of their loved ones. Herron closed its doors in November.

Peter Wheeland said he had little interest in all the promises of investigation—he was preoccupied with caring for his mom. The nurses who came into the home reported that she was not well, but provincial policy was to not test residents but, rather, to behave as if everyone was potentially infected. Another provincial directive stated that residents of long-term-care homes should not be transferred to hospital unless they were gravely ill, and in many cases physicians advised that they would be better off getting comfort care or palliative care at the homes.

Peter Wheeland balked at the bureaucratic rules and insisted his mother be transferred to hospital, where she tested positive for Covid-19. Even though she had a relatively mild case, "she was in horrible shape, she refused to eat or drink, and suffered delirium." But she eventually recovered and, according to Peter, "there was no way in hell she was going back to Herron."

The family decided instead to rent an apartment and care for their mother with a combination of family caregiving and home care services. Despite her significant health problems—her severe arthritis leaves her largely immobile—she was granted just one hour of home care daily, with thirty minutes in the morning and thirty more in the evening, and the loan of a hospital bed and lift. That was supplemented with three hours daily of home care services purchased from a private agency, and her children took turns living with and caring for her the rest of the time. This routine continued for several months while Connie was on the wait list for a long-term-care home in Ontario, near her daughter.

Peter Wheeland says the family's greatest regret is that they didn't consider home care earlier. "I realize now that my parents' needs could have easily been met at home for many years. But no one ever offered that possibility; they were constantly pushed toward institutional care."

At one point, that care, which ended up being second-rate, was costing $110,000 a year. "Surely, for that kind of money, we could have done a lot better," he says.

Surprisingly, Wheeland is not particularly bitter towards Herron. "I think it was happenstance that my parents were at Herron and that it ended up getting a lot of press," he says. "The truth is, what happened there happened everywhere. It was awful, but it certainly wasn't unique."

He's right about that.

While the government reacted to the Herron mess with strong words and promises to get the outbreak under control, the coronavirus continued to spread in residential care homes, the death count climbed steadily, and staffing shortages became worse. Ontario experienced a similarly gloomy trifecta of problems, and public outrage grew. At the end of April, Quebec's premier asked for help from the Canadian Forces, and Ontario followed suit.

The sight of camouflage-clad soldiers coming to the rescue of elders was a striking one that underscored just how grave the situation had become. They were deployed to twenty-eight of the hardest-hit facilities in Quebec and five in Ontario. The soldiers—most of them physicians, nurses, physician assistants and care aides—went about their business quietly and efficiently. But after they left, they dropped a bombshell: a 21-page memo to the Minister of National Defence outlining what they had witnessed in the Ontario facilities. "We identified a number of medical and professional issues present," Brigadier-General C.J.J. Mialkowski wrote with Churchillian understatement. Some of the "observations" included:

- residents who had not been bathed in weeks
- patients left in soiled incontinence pads and beds
- little or no turning of patients, leading to pressure ulcers
- reusing of non-sterile supplies such as catheters, syringes and intravenous lines
- lack of pain treatment, including a patient with a fractured hip and inadequate palliation
- aggressive behaviour, including forceful feeding causing audible choking/aspiration

- residents going hungry to the point where soldiers felt it necessary to share their personal food
- insect infestation, including ants and cockroaches.

A second report about the state of Quebec homes came to similar conclusions, with slightly more muted language. In short, the Canadian Forces, with its outsider's perspective, reminded the public that abuse and neglect were happening on a grand scale in institutional care.

After months of lockdown, the spread of coronavirus eventually slowed in long-term-care and nursing homes. But it's hard to overstate just how lethal the outbreaks proved to be. Nora Loreto, a journalist and activist based in Quebec City, meticulously mapped all the deaths in long-term-care facilities across Canada during the pandemic, and the data she compiled is mind-numbingly depressing.

As of September 30, Canada had recorded 9,262 Covid-19 deaths, and of that total, 7,609 were in residential care homes. That's 82 percent—twice the average in the thirty-seven OECD countries (of which Canada is one). Loreto identified cases in 670 facilities with at least one Covid-19 death. The top fifty hardest hit:

FACILITY	CITY	PROV.	DEATHS	# OF BEDS
CHSLD Vigi Mont-Royal	Montreal	QC	102	273
Centre d'hébergement Sainte-Dorothée	Laval	QC	101	285
Centre d'hébergement Notre-Dame-de-la-Merci	Montreal	QC	100	398
CHSLD Laurendeau	Montreal	QC	93	300

FACILITY	CITY	PROV.	DEATHS	# OF BEDS
Centre d'hébergement Champlain–Marie-Victorin	Montreal	QC	85	280
CHSLD Yvon-Brunet	Montreal	QC	77	185
CHSLD Vigi Dollard-des-Ormeaux	Dollard-des-Ormeaux	QC	74	160
CHSLD Saint-Jude	Laval	QC	73	204
Camilla Care Community	Mississauga	ON	72	237
Orchard Villa LTC	Pickering	ON	70	233
CHSLD Pierre-Joseph-Triest	Montreal	QC	69	227
CHSLD Grace Dart	Montreal	QC	69	94
CHSLD Angelica	Montreal	QC	67	350
Centre d'hébergement Jean-De La Lande	Montreal	QC	65	276
CHSLD Joseph-François-Perreault	Montreal	QC	64	192
Downsview Long Term Care Centre	North York	ON	64	252
Résidence Berthiaume-Du Tremblay	Montreal	QC	63	198
Carlingview Manor	Ottawa	ON	61	303
Résidence Herron	Dorval	QC	61	139
Villa Val des Arbres	Laval	QC	60	145
Centre d'hébergement de Lachine	Lachine	QC	59	n/a

FACILITY	CITY	PROV.	DEATHS	# OF BEDS
L'Institut universitaire de gériatrie de Montréal	Montreal	QC	57	446
Centre d'hébergement de LaSalle	LaSalle	QC	55	202
Centre d'hébergement René-Lévesque	Longeuil	QC	55	224
CHSLD Jean-Hubert-Biermans	Montreal	QC	55	203
CHSLD Benjamin-Victor-Rousselot	Montreal	QC	54	157
Centre d'hébergement Cloutier-du Rivage	Trois Rivières	QC	53	179
Centre d'hébergement l'Éden de Laval	Laval	QC	53	152
Altamont Care Community	Scarborough	ON	53	159
Northwood Manor	Halifax	NS	53	485
Forest Heights Revera	Waterloo	ON	51	240
CHSLD Jeanne-Le Ber	Montreal	QC	50	351
Madonna Care Community	Orleans	ON	49	160
Extendicare Guildwood	Scarborough	ON	48	169
Hawthorne Place Care Centre	North York	ON	48	269
Isabel and Arthur Meighen Manor	Toronto	ON	48	168
CHSLD Auclair	Montreal	QC	45	160
CHSLD de Saint-Laurent	Montreal	QC	45	n/a

FACILITY	CITY	PROV.	DEATHS	# OF BEDS
Centre multiservices de santé et de services sociaux Laflèche	Shawinigan	QC	44	154
CHSLD la Pinière	Laval	QC	42	100
CHSLD de la Rive	Laval	QC	42	94
Centre d'hébergement des Seigneurs	Montreal	QC	42	168
Eatonville Care Centre	Etobicoke	ON	42	247
Midland Gardens Care Community	Scarborough	ON	42	299
Jardins du Haut Saint-Laurent	Saint-Augustin-de-Desmaures	QC	41	n/a
Seven Oaks	Scarborough	ON	41	249
CHSLD Hope	Montreal	QC	40	160
CHSLD Paul-Lizotte	Montreal	QC	40	128
Jeffery Hale / Saint Brigid's	Quebec City	QC	40	99
Centre Hospitalier Gériatrique Maimonides	Côte St-Luc	QC	39	387

In terms of deaths, Résidence Herron ties for sixteenth. Another noteworthy entry, even though it ranks much lower: Lynn Valley in North Vancouver.

On March 7, 2020, Dr. Bonnie Henry, British Columbia's Provincial Health Officer, announced that there was an outbreak of coronavirus at Lynn Valley Care Centre, a 204-bed private long-term-care facility. At one point in a seemingly routine press conference, where she announced that two residents had been infected, she was overcome by emotion.

Dr. Henry, a veteran of the Canadian navy and countless public health battles, both domestic and international, is tough as nails. Her response was telling. "This is one of the scenarios that we have been, of course, most concerned about," she said in what turned out to be a remarkable understatement. She was fighting back tears, she said, because she couldn't help but imagine the pain families were feeling at the news.

A novel respiratory virus infiltrating a facility that is full of seniors who are frail and suffering from chronic illnesses is a nightmare scenario. Worse still, it looked as though a health care worker had carried the bug into the home. In an added wrinkle, the worker appeared to have been infected in the community, making it the first Canadian case that was not travel-related. The day after Dr. Henry's emotional press conference, one of the infected residents, a man in his 80s, died. It was the first death in a long-term-care facility in Canada. The circumstances of that death set off alarm bells.

"Seniors who live in seniors' homes are intrinsically more at risk of infectious diseases," says Dr. Roger Wong, a clinical professor of geriatric medicine at the University of British Columbia. It is their underlying health conditions, including dementia, cardiovascular disease and chronic obstructive pulmonary disease (COPD), that make them more vulnerable, especially as the immune system weakens with age. Even at the best of times, residents are easy prey for microbes. Influenza and pneumonia kill hundreds, sometimes thousands, of seniors in Canada each year, despite extensive vaccination campaigns. Gastroenteritis outbreaks caused by bugs such as norovirus are commonplace even with the best infection control measures. Adding a novel coronavirus to the mix posed an even greater challenge.

Dr. Henry recognized that protecting residents meant limiting their contact with other people. But care homes see a steady stream of visitors, including many family members who are there every single day for years. The facilities also employ a lot of staff, many of whom work part-time and at multiple homes. (At least one-third of care aides in Canada have more than one job.) Four days after the Lynn Valley outbreak, another case was detected at Hollyburn House Retirement Residence in West Vancouver. The same worker had done shifts at both facilities, and was the likely carrier.

As soon as the first outbreak was detected, Dr. Henry ordered Lynn Valley to implement more stringent infection control measures, including requiring workers with flu-like symptoms to stay home and isolating any resident who seemed sick. In addition, all workers were required to have PPE, which had been mandatory in all hospitals but not in care homes.

Regarding sick days, workers in many homes not only were denied them but were actually ordered to work even if they were sick. (The reasons so many workers are employed on a part-time basis is so employers can avoid paying benefits like sick days. Every day staying home sick costs workers dearly, many of whom are scraping by on wages as low as $13 an hour.) As for isolating sick residents, it was often physically impossible. Most care homes are old and built like hospitals, with many having three or four beds to a room, with just curtains separating them, and residents using communal bathrooms and dining halls.

Dr. Henry banned all visitors, acknowledging this would be a hardship because family caregivers provide a lot of essential support, and because further isolation would be detrimental to residents' mental health. Soon after, she would outlaw the common practice of nurses and care aides working in more than one facility. Further, she used the Provincial Health Officer's extensive powers to take over staffing in all of BC's care homes to ensure the rules were strictly followed.

There is no doubt the swift and decisive action by Dr. Henry saved lives. By September 2020, BC had recorded just 140 deaths in care facilities. Quebec and Ontario, both of which dithered before moving to protect seniors in care, had recorded more than 4,600 and 2,800 deaths respectively. (And bear in mind, these are likely underestimates. Ontario, for example, doesn't track deaths in retirement homes.) It was mid-March when BC asked staff to stop working in multiple facilities; two weeks later, it was made an official order. Ontario moved to forbid staff from working at multiple homes only two weeks after that, whereas Quebec has still not outlawed the practice, despite the fact that, in Montreal alone, more than 5,500 workers tested positive.

Because of the SARS experience, it became a priority for individual institutions, as well as provincial and federal officials, to ensure that hospitals would be prepared to respond to the pandemic. Long-term-care facilities, nursing homes and other institutions that house seniors at high risk were seemingly forgotten, in large part because they are not part of the medicare system—and the price for that oversight proved high.

Dr. Henry said one of the reasons she was so deeply concerned by the Lynn Valley situation was related to what was going on just across the border, in Washington State. At that time, a highly publicized coronavirus outbreak was tearing through the Life Care Center in Kirkland, Washington; sixteen residents in the 120-bed suburban Seattle facility had already died of Covid-19, dozens more were infected, and many staff members were showing symptoms. (The final death toll at Life Care was thirty-seven.)

There was no doubt that one case of Covid-19 in a seniors' facility could quickly set off a wildfire of infection and death.

Despite the early warnings, the response in most jurisdictions—BC being the exception—was slow and tepid. What happened at Herron, and hundreds of other institutions entrusted with the care of our loved ones, is troubling, sickening and, in many cases, verging on criminal. But all those deaths, all that suffering, were not caused by Covid-19 alone. The wily coronavirus merely preyed on a system that left residents vulnerable, on public policies that have long neglected elders, and on a culture where, after a certain age, you cease to have value to society.

Covid-19 exposed a long-standing truth: we have failed what is often called "the greatest generation," those who survived the Great Depression and the Second World War. And we're on track to fail their children too, the baby boomers, unless we act swiftly and decisively to fix eldercare in this country.

CHAPTER 2

Prisoner of History

Belmont House, located in Toronto's tony Yorkville neighbourhood, calls itself the "Seniors' Home of Choice." The spacious grounds feature spectacular gardens, including an enclosed rooftop garden designed to allow people with dementia to wander safely. Antique furniture, fireside lounges, spacious dining rooms, and well-appointed private and semi-private rooms all exude a sense of comfort, the antithesis of how institutional care is perceived by the public.

But it was not always so. The history of Belmont House is a microcosm of how eldercare has evolved in Canada, providing a glimpse of its past, its present and perhaps even its future.

It began in 1852 with a small group of Anglican Church women. At the time, Toronto was a bustling city of thirty thousand, and the residents were almost exclusively British. The city had a women's prison but no facilities resembling the modern halfway house for women once they were released. The charitable church ladies decided to rent a home downtown and create a private institution to care for the former prisoners, most of whom had been arrested, convicted without trial and jailed for undesirable social behaviours such as promiscuity or having a child out of wedlock. By 1860 more space was required, so the Christian charity purchased a 3.5-acre lot that included a large farmhouse. In 1873 a larger home was built on site and given a formal name: Magdalene Asylum and Industrial House of Refuge.

Asylums and houses of refuge were patterned after British workhouses, and the inmates/residents were often subjected to hard labour, rigid rules, poor food, overcrowding and suboptimal living conditions. Conditions at the Magdalene facility may have been slightly less grim because, at homes run by Christian charities, residents were admitted of their own free will rather than committed involuntarily. But the name is a reminder that our institutional eldercare has its origins in the penal system, not the health system.

For centuries, the poor were treated as the authors of their own misfortune. The philosophy was codified in the Elizabethan Poor Laws of 1601, which were the basis of social welfare programs for more than 250 years. The legislation essentially stated that the marginalized of society should be taken care of, but there should be no handouts, and certainly no pampering. The poor were classified in two broad categories: 1) the "impotent poor" who could not look after themselves, which included the very old, the very young, the sick, the crippled, unmarried mothers, the blind and the insane; and 2) the "able-bodied" poor who had no work and no money to live on. The second group was treated with more disdain than the first, but the institutionalized poor, regardless of their age or physical abilities, were largely considered inmates who had to work for their keep and should receive only the bare minimum of sustenance.

Workhouses were transplanted to Upper Canada by British settlers, and housed criminals, the poor, orphans and the elderly rather indiscriminately. Over time, however, these institutions became more specialized, designated as "gaols" (penitentiaries), lunatic asylums, orphanages, homes for unwed mothers and homes for the aged. The latter had names like "home for the friendless," "aged women's home" and "house of refuge."

By 1883, the Magdalene Asylum was a house of refuge and had grown so large that it had separate buildings for older women and older men. In 1890 the sprawling group of buildings was renamed Belmont House, and accommodated more than 250 residents aged 65 to 90. In addition to the charitable cases, some spots were sold to families who wanted to house their elderly parents or grandparents, and they were given preferential treatment. The institution had trouble keeping up with demand.

"We have this romantic notion that seniors were beloved and revered, but the reality is that their lives were often harsh, not romantic," says Lisa Levin, CEO of AdvantAge Ontario, a group that was founded more than a century ago as the Association of Managers of Homes for the Aged and Infirm. There were a surprisingly large number of these homes, funded mostly by municipalities and religious orders, but Levin notes that the residents were essentially forced to work, and even wore uniforms like prisoners.

The workhouse model existed until well after the Second World War. The welfare state that developed in the postwar years would usher in more compassionate care for the disadvantaged. In 1946, Ontario appointed its first inspector of houses of refuge. L.E. Ludlow, a principled civil servant and larger-than-life character, set out to single-handedly reshape the Dickensian homes into comfortable facilities that cared for elders rather than worked them to death.

The province adopted the Homes for the Aged Act, setting out some basic standards and providing about one-third of the funding to houses of refuge, giving the government leverage to demand change. Ludlow wanted to end forced labour and common practices like solitary confinement for rule breakers, and during his tenure he made tremendous progress. He railed about things he witnessed during his inspections, such as an elderly woman on her hands and knees scrubbing floors, and a white-haired man locked in a basement cell because he had dared to talk during a meal. Ludlow also lobbied to get municipalities to build better facilities, dragging councillors along to the worst homes, where they witnessed "conditions so deplorable they retched." He also noted that some places that were funded by religious groups had fewer institutional aspects and were more like real homes, and decided that type of setting should be the norm.

When Ludlow left the post of inspector of homes of refuge in 1961, the transformation of residential care for the elderly was well under way, not only in Ontario but around the country, where there was a hodgepodge of public, private and charitable homes; quality and standards varied tremendously, and abuse and financial exploitation were rampant. In Ludlow's final report, he recommended new legislation that, for example, would outlaw forced labour (this regulation came into effect several years later) and limit rooms to four beds (this still hasn't happened, six decades later). After he left office, Ludlow would say he had really wanted the limit to be two beds per room, but he knew that would be considered spendthrift and decadent and never be accepted at a time when wards with twenty beds were not uncommon.

In 1966, Ontario adopted the Nursing Home Act. There was not only new terminology but also a dramatically different philosophy. Elders would not work for their keep anymore; they would be cared for lovingly. According to Lisa Levin, that's when care homes got dramatically better. "People went to nursing homes voluntarily and eagerly. It was a place where you would drink tea out of china cups, play bingo and golf, and enjoy a comfortable retirement."

This kind of transformation was happening everywhere. Belmont House, like many other former homes of refuge, undertook an extensive expansion and rebuilding project.

In the period between Confederation and Expo in 1967 and the 1976 Montreal Olympics, no dream was too big, no project too ambitious. Many billions of dollars were spent, mostly on new infrastructure, including hospitals, schools, hockey arenas, public housing and libraries, as well as nursing homes and long-term-care facilities. Quebec alone built sixty thousand new spots in long-term-care facilities (CHSLDs). "The homes were well-funded. People were well-lodged, well-fed and even entertained," says Jean-Pierre Lavoie, a social gerontologist and professor at the Université du Québec à Montréal. While the homes were designed to care for people with chronic illnesses, most of the residents were in relatively good health, to the point where it is said that the parking lots of nursing homes emptied every winter as the resident snowbirds headed to Florida.

All these investments in improving the health of the young and old alike made it feel as though Canada was growing up and taking its place on the world stage. And of course, this golden era had kicked off two decades earlier with the boldest initiative of all: universal public health care.

Publicly funded health insurance had its beginnings in Saskatchewan in 1947, when Premier Tommy Douglas introduced hospital insurance. Hospital insurance was designed principally to help families avoid crippling debts from hospital stays for acute illness and injury. At the time, Canada was still very much a rural nation. Infectious diseases like polio affected a lot of children, many women suffered pregnancy- and childbirth-related harms, and men fell prey to traumatic injuries at factories and farms, and often could not afford care.

Another driving force behind medicare, and one that is often overlooked, was the care of veterans. Unlike other Canadians, soldiers and former soldiers who had served overseas were eligible for medical care at no charge. The federal Department of Veterans Affairs operated eleven hospitals across the country, with almost eight thousand beds in total, as well as rehabilitation centres and long-term-care homes for veterans of the First World War. But there was tremendous political pressure to extend the benefits enjoyed by soldiers to their families and the general public.

Universal hospital insurance became a national program in 1957 when the federal government adopted the Hospital Insurance and Diagnostic Services Act. Ottawa agreed to reimburse the provinces 50 percent of spending on hospital care and diagnostics (such as X-rays and a brand new technology, ultrasound). There were two conditions for provinces to receive funds from the federal government: 1) access must be universal, meaning no one would be refused care based on inability to pay; and 2) there would be no user fees, meaning hospital care would be "free."

In 1962, Saskatchewan again became a trailblazer, expanding its provincial insurance program to cover physician services. A few years later, in 1966, Ottawa followed suit again, adopting the Medical Care Act, agreeing to cover 50 percent of physician services, with the provinces covering the balance. To receive the money, provinces needed to respect the same conditions as for hospital funding: universality and no user fees. That's when the term "medicare" (which was the name given to a similar insurance program for seniors in the US) became the norm. And that's what medicare is to this day: public funding of hospital and physician services contingent on respecting some basic principles.

One of the consequences of universal health insurance was that veterans no longer required special treatment, so the large network of military hospitals, including Sunnybrook Hospital in Toronto, was transferred to the provinces, with a proviso that veterans would get priority treatment, especially for long-term care. In retrospect, this was a big mistake. If Canada had continued to fund stand-alone facilities for veterans as they grew older (which is an easy political sell), those facilities could have become the cornerstone of a much-needed long-term-care system.

There were vague plans—perhaps "dreams" is a better descriptor—to extend medicare to other aspects of medical care, such as prescription drugs, home care services and dental care. But LTC didn't get a lot of consideration, for two principal reasons: it was seen more as a housing issue than a health issue, and it was believed the hospital system would provide all the care elders required.

In fact, long-term care has long wallowed, largely neglected at the intersection of housing, social welfare and health. Many ministries had a claim to it, but none really had responsibility, at least until recently. Up until now, Canada has largely left LTC in the purview of families. In many Western countries, it was never really part of the mainstream welfare state. The exceptions were Nordic countries such as Norway and Sweden, which began funding universal programs for eldercare in the 1940s, at the same time as universal health care.

But things got complicated in the 1960s and 1970s. Driven by the women's liberation movement and economic necessity, women were entering the workforce in large numbers and were less willing and able to care for their parents and grandparents at home. There was an exodus from rural to urban areas as families and workers became more mobile. As a result, people became increasingly distanced from their extended families.

At the same time, the deinstitutionalization movement, fuelled by a combination of civil rights demands and cost-cutting initiatives, meant that psychiatric facilities were being shuttered. In 1960, Canada had more than sixty thousand psychiatric beds, compared with six thousand today—and the country's population has since doubled. These institutions housed patients with severe illnesses like schizophrenia, but also many older people with dementia, who ended up in hospitals when they were deinstitutionalized.

Hospitals, in turn, were faced with new pressures. There were dramatic medical advances in that period, with the development of effective treatments for cancer and heart disease, and science fiction–like ideas such as organ transplantation became a reality. Not only were these technological innovations expensive, but they accelerated the transformation of hospitals. Temples of healing—hospitals—date back to ancient Greece. But for millennia they were largely places people went to die, where the only real care offered was prayer. That was true, at least in part, well into the twentieth century. But as medicine progressed, especially with the advent of the antibiotic era, hospitals saw the number of acute-care patients skyrocket. Not only were there more surgeries, but everyday activities like childbirth became medicalized, especially after the Second World War, so beds were at a premium. The days of elderly patients spending their final weeks and months in a hospital bed, cared for by nurses, were coming to an end.

Most importantly of all, the demographics of Canada were beginning to change quite dramatically. So too were political priorities as the baby boomers grew up. As the Senate Committee on Aging noted: "Canada has become pre-occupied with maternal and child health to the exclusion of other age groups." In 1960, less than 8 percent of the population was over the age of 65, while young people under the age of 15 were far more numerous, at 34 percent.

Elders were still respected; after all, they were the generation that had survived the Great War. But boom times had left them behind. Families were caring for their own less and less, and private pensions were still rare. Before the creation of the Canada Pension Plan in 1965, more than one in four seniors lived in poverty—often abject poverty. The CPP, which paid the equivalent of 25 percent of a worker's average lifetime salary annually, left the beneficiaries only marginally better off. In addition, when the CPP was created and the retirement age set at sixty-five, life expectancy in Canada was only 67.

While there was enthusiastic interest and investment in infrastructure, and all the ribbon-cutting opportunities new buildings created for politicians, there was a lot less focus on program funding. Nursing homes and long-term-care facilities were being built, but many elders could not afford to live in them. The housing component was paid privately, and government subsidies were available only for the "indigent," the poorest of the poor. But even for those with some retirement savings, the minimum out-of-pocket costs, $8 to $10 a day for the most basic accommodation in a four-bed ward room, could still be out of reach. Increasingly, priority was given to clients with serious health conditions. Senior care facilities like CHSLDs became less welcoming and homelike and more like hospitals, but without the staffing and funding hospitals were afforded by medicare.

In the 1970s, health costs were soaring, routinely increasing by more than 10 percent per annum, even as services were cut, thanks to double-digit inflation. The emphasis was on reining in spending, not expanding medicare. One of the few politicians pushing for medicare to cover eldercare (both LTC and home care) was Tommy Douglas, who, after his government was defeated in Saskatchewan, became a federal member of Parliament. "A lot could be done in this country by the establishment of more nursing homes, the provision of home-care treatment, meals on wheels, more extended care units in hospitals," he said in the House of Commons. But the pleas of the father of medicare were largely ignored. In Douglas's words, "a great silence loomed over residential care for seniors."

In fact, there was a long period of ad hoc-ism. Governments, federal and provincial, would have brief bursts of enthusiasm for eldercare—usually just before an election, when they were jockeying for the votes of seniors—and then quickly lose interest. For example, in the early 1970s the federal government created the Extended Health Care Services program, offering provinces $20 per capita to bolster eldercare, an amount that grew over time. But the money came with no strings attached, so it ended up going into the provinces' general health spending, where it was gobbled up by hospitals.

A watershed moment for medicare occurred in 1984, the year Health Minister Monique Bégin tabled legislation creating the Canada Health Act. The bill set out the five conditions provinces were required to meet in order to receive health dollars from the federal government. Those preconditions, all of which already existed in legislation and regulations, came to be viewed as the principles defining modern Canadian medicare:

1. *Public administration*: Provincial health insurance programs must be publicly accountable for the funds they spend, and administered by a not-for-profit authority.
2. *Accessibility*: Canadians must have reasonable access to insured services without charge or paying user fees.
3. *Comprehensiveness*: Provincial health insurance programs must cover all medically necessary services.

4. *Universality*: No one will be denied care because of an inability to pay, and user fees are not permitted for medically necessary care.

5. *Portability*: Canadians are covered by a provincial insurance plan regardless of where they live, even during short absences from their province of residence.

Two of the key words in the legislation are "medically necessary." Those words apply to medical procedures and treatments paid for by provincial health insurance plans, meaning hospital care and physician services. Under the Canada Health Act, long-term care was not deemed medically necessary. Nor were home care, prescription drugs, vision care, hearing aids, physiotherapy and many other health services that are covered by public insurance programs in other countries. The legislation makes passing mention of "adult residential care service" and "nursing home intermediate service" being part of "extended health care services," but these terms were never defined in the all-important regulations related to the act, and so they fell by the wayside.

After the legislative snub, eldercare became, arguably, even more marginalized. The Canadian Medical Association, which created a Task Force on Allocation of Health Care Resources in 1985 to examine the impacts of the Canada Health Act, called the lack of federal funding for LTC and home care "social negligence." The CMA was particularly critical of the lack of investment in government-owned and not-for-profit care homes, saying elders were being left at the mercy of for-profit corporations.

In the years that followed, as it became clear public funding would stagnate, for-profit homes expanded appreciably. So did neglect. Eldercare largely fell off the political and public policy radar.

Only a small group of dedicated researchers seemed to be paying attention, and their attempts to sound the alarm went unheeded. "Long-term residential care was largely invisible in Canadian policy debates," says Pat Armstrong, a Canadian sociologist and distinguished research professor at York University.

In the late 1990s, however, at least in the province of Quebec, journalists took up the cause. André Noël, an investigative reporter at Montreal's *La Presse*, wrote a series of jaw-dropping articles exposing how more than four hundred elders had died of neglect in Quebec long-term-care facilities. The *Journal de Montréal* routinely had headlines like NO BATH FOR TWO YEARS. The scrutiny of the press led to coroner's inquiries, public inquiries and government reports, all of which detailed the failings in LTC.

Next came regulation, lots and lots of new rules—but not much more funding. Whether public, not-for-profit or private, homes had their rates set by government edict. But the funding often made it near impossible to deliver the care required. Homes cut where it was easiest; the largest budget item, by far, is labour. Skilled nurses were cut to make way for less skilled and lower-paid care aides. Patient loads increased. Shifts were shortened so workers would take care of more patients in a shorter time. Union contracts were torn up and wages and benefits were cut.

Meanwhile, the average age of the clientele at care homes was climbing and, consequently, residents were more frail; the number of patients with dementia and multiple chronic illnesses skyrocketed. Demographics again. When the aging of baby boomers began to be described as a "grey tsunami," it was very much a misnomer. A tsunami is a sudden, violent, unexpected wave that takes people by surprise; the baby boomers getting older was entirely predictable for about half a century. The problem we have in Canada is not an aging society, which is actually a triumph of medicine and social policy. The problem is that we have done so little to prepare.

The baby boom coincided with some tremendous scientific advances and economic and social changes that resulted in life expectancy soaring and fertility dropping. Gen-Xers, more educated and socially mobile than their parents (and with the advantage of readily available birth control), had far fewer children, and had them later in life, and millennials are becoming parents even later still.

This lower fertility rate is an important factor in the future of eldercare. Canadian women, on average, have 1.5 babies, well below the replacement rate of 2.1. If it were not for immigration, Canada's population would be declining. As it is, the demographic makeup of the country is changing markedly. For the first time in history, there are more people in Canada over the age of 65 than under the age of 14. By 2050, it is projected that there will be twice as many seniors as children and youth. Where will the workforce come from to care for elders? With a shrinking tax base, how will we pay for the growing cost of care?

Life expectancy at birth in Canada in 1945 was 68 for women and 65 for men. Today, it is 84 for women and 80 for men. Even more striking is life expectancy once a person reaches 65. After the Second World War, a Canadian could expect their "golden years" (those after 65) to last 13 years; today, it is 21 years on average. Those extra years have another notable characteristic: most are not disability-free. At least half of new retirees will live past 85, or to "senior-senior" status, and most of them will have severe physical and mental disabilities, which has implications for everything from pensions and LTC to how we design municipalities.

The most striking reality about the senior-senior population is the rate of dementia. Aging itself doesn't cause dementia, but by age 85 almost one-third of elders have the neurological condition, and almost half of that segment end up in institutional care. As a result, the vast majority of long-term-care residents now have dementia, along with a multitude of other health conditions. But care homes were not built with this clientele in mind, nor have workers been trained specifically to deal with their needs. Furthermore, funding has not been adjusted to reflect the fact that caring for dementia patients requires much more time and effort.

The challenge of caring for that cohort of senior-seniors is only going to grow. The oldest of the baby boomers will turn 75 in 2021, and the fastest-growing demographic group are centenarians. In nursing homes and long-term-care homes, hundredth-birthday parties, which used to be big news, are now commonplace.

We also can't forget that the large majority of elders are relatively healthy. According to Statistics Canada, 20 percent of those over the age of 65 describe their health as fair, bad or very bad—but that means 80 percent consider their health to be good or very good. However, as time marches on, most elders will eventually need some form of long-term care.

Demographic data is often viewed as abstract, even trivial. But we can't improve eldercare unless we have a good grasp on who it is intended to serve, what their needs are and what kind of workforce is required, as well as what financial investments must be made to provide that care—not just today but in the future. Too often we use data to tell us, in retrospect, where we have failed; we should be using it to tell us how to plan and how to take action. Currently, in Canada, only 11 percent of LTC is provided at home, the other 89 percent in institutions (7 percent in hospitals, 82 percent in nursing homes and long-term-care facilities.) Most Western countries, especially those with particularly good eldercare, such as Denmark and Sweden, have been steadily decreasing institutional care for decades and placing the emphasis on care in the community. We have to decide where that care can and should be provided.

It's almost as if the treatment of elders has come close to full circle over the past century and a half. The paupers, Canadians with no pensions and savings, aren't subjected to forced labour anymore, but they get only the bare minimum, such as a spot in a four-bed ward room and a couple of hours of hands-on care daily. That sort of relegation to second-class status was supposed to have ended with medicare and its grand principle that no one would be denied care because of an inability to pay. But medicare, paradoxically, created two classes of care: hospitals and doctors funded universally, and everything else funded largely through private payment.

"We build university hospitals for billions of dollars and we don't have places for our elders to live," says André-Pierre Contandriopoulos, professor emeritus in the Department of Public Health at the Université de Montréal. "It's unacceptable."

CHAPTER 3

Long-Term Carelessness

The moral test of government is how it treats those who are
in the dawn of life, the children; those who are in the twilight
of life, the aged; and those in the shadows of life, the needy
and the handicapped.

HUBERT H. HUMPHREY, 1977

Before the coronavirus pandemic, not many Canadian elders were
keen about the idea of ending up in a long-term-care home. By late
2020, after more than 10,000 Covid-19 deaths in institutional care in
under a year, the emotions of most have shifted from ambivalence
to genuine fear. Their children also are experiencing heightened
dread about reaching the point where they can no longer provide
assistance and LTC appears to be the only option left.

Fearful of care. Guilty about needing help. How did it come to
this in a country that takes so much pride in its health system?

"We failed them. We broke the covenant," a blue-ribbon panel
appointed by the Royal Society of Canada said in a report published in June 2020. While that comment was ostensibly about the
Covid-19 crisis in care homes, the experts made it clear that the

failure was much broader, and the response had to be as well. "We have a duty, a responsibility and the ability to fix this—not just to fix the current communicable disease crisis, but to fix the sector that helped wreak such avoidable and tragic havoc."

Covid-19 did not break the long-term-care system, the panel said. Rather, it was a shock wave that exposed an already broken system, one with "longstanding, widespread and pervasive deficiencies." Surprisingly, their damning report concluded on a positive note: "We can restore trust."

But where to begin? Canada's elders are the primary beneficiaries of the health and social welfare systems. But those once-robust social programs, most created when the boomers were just babies, are outdated and rickety. If the growing cohort of seniors is going to age with grace and dignity, much needs to be done to provide better primary care, more accessible home care, better housing, more senior-friendly communities, more support for caregivers, better income supports, and policy changes that address deeply ingrained ageism. But, clearly, the highest priority for reform is where the carnage occurred on an unprecedented scale: in institutional care. Before we can fix it, though, we need to understand the system and its failings.

The good news—if we dare state it in that manner—is that every problem has been exposed repeatedly and in painful detail. Since the advent of medicare, there have been countless examinations of the inadequacies of eldercare. Politicians have been far more eager to order investigations than act on the problems that have been exposed.

More shocking than the sheer number of reports is their remarkable consistency. The same failings are underlined time and time again:

- Institutional care is more industrial than personal. The priority is always building more beds, not providing better care.
- Care homes are not homes as much as pseudo-hospitals with a much lower level of care than actual hospitals.
- The care people need in the final years and months of their lives is complex and costly, but we keep trying to deliver it on the cheap.
- The infrastructure is terribly outdated. Homes are designed and built for assembly line efficiency, not for comfort.
- Staffing is grossly inadequate and getting worse with each passing year as the complexity of residents' needs grows and staff turnover is astronomical, about 25 percent annually.
- Sending frail elders to LTC is the default. It's the first choice when it should be the last resort.
- Unlike medical care, long-term care is neither universally accessible nor affordable to all, a reality that undermines the philosophy of medicare.
- Infection control is poor. Oversight is lax. Standards are few. Quality is not rewarded.
- No one is ultimately responsible for ensuring elders get the care they need in a timely, accessible fashion.
- Families are conflicted beyond belief about how best to care for their loved ones, and the system doesn't make the choices clear or easy.

"The challenge we have is twofold: 1) Who needs to be in long-term care? and 2) How do we care appropriately for those who really need to be there?" says Dr. Samir Sinha, director of geriatrics at Sinai Health System and University Health Network in Toronto. He believes the first question is relatively simple to answer, at least in theory. Long-term care should be reserved for those who need constant monitoring, such as patients with advanced dementia, and for people whose care needs exceed what their family can provide.

Dr. Sinha treats people with complex care needs who are in their 80s, 90s and 100s, and his patients, almost universally, want to remain at home as they age. But they don't want to be a burden, nor do they want to be alone, so they often ask if they should be in long-term care. "To answer them, I have a formula. I say: 'Do you have family that can take care of you?' and 'Do you have money?' If you're a senior in this country, those are the two elements that will determine your future."

Mary Huang, an Ottawa engineer, got to the point where her two parents needed to be in LTC, but she said it was a heart-wrenching decision. "It's really, really difficult to put your parents in a home, especially if you're from the Chinese culture. We respect and care for our elders," she says.

Like many caregivers, Mary made superhuman efforts to keep her parents at home, and did so for almost five years before institutional care became necessary. (Her two siblings pitched in but didn't have as much flexibility.) Her mother, Anna Huang, had a heart attack in 2013, at age 81, and over the years the health challenges piled up: pancreatitis, hearing loss, severe anemia, vascular dementia and more. Her father, Peter Huang, had a similar journey, but his decline was even more rapid: a heart attack in 2014 at age 88, followed by gall bladder removal, vascular dementia, a stroke and so on.

As Anna's and Peter's health issues increased, there were regular stints in the hospital, followed by home care. At one point there were personal support workers (PSWs) coming to the home six days a week. The help was welcome but not always reliable, and it required a lot of organization and oversight on daughter Mary's part.

When her father began to wander, as many dementia patients do, it was time to sell the family home and move into a more secure location. "My mom said we had to get more doors between Dad and the outside," Mary recalls. They decided to purchase a condo where there would be an extra room for a live-in caregiver. Mary was also going to purchase a separate condo in the same building so she could be nearby to help. "I'm an engineer, I have an MBA, a great career, and I travel the world, but I dropped everything to care for my parents," she said. "That's what was expected of me."

In August 2017, Peter Huang had a stroke and his cognition diminished noticeably. Condo living was no longer feasible. He spent the next sixteen months in the Ottawa Hospital as an "alternate level of care" patient, waiting for a spot in a long-term-care home.

Mary found the wait very long and stressful. "They kept pressuring us to take any bed that was available, but there was no way." She had done her homework, conducting extensive research, visiting numerous long-term-care homes and even approaching random family members outside care facilities to ask them questions. "Most of them were glad to help," Mary says. If there is one thing every family knows, it is that practical information is hard to come by.

When her father finally got a placement, in December 2018, at the Glebe Centre in Ottawa, it was a perfect fit. "He's on the Chinese floor and that's really important because he's losing his English," Mary says. The building is only a decade old, the staffing ratio is good at one PSW per eight patients during the day, there are a lot of activities, and the staff is engaged. "Everything on my checklist," Mary says.

While Peter was in hospital, Anna moved into a retirement home, but her plans changed too. After a lengthy hospitalization for a blood disorder, she joined Peter at the Glebe Centre. However, the couple live in separate rooms on different floors, for practical reasons: almost all the patients on the Chinese floor have advanced dementia, but Mrs. Huang is healthier and much more sociable, so it would not be a good fit.

The family home was sold and the roughly $300,000 the sale netted was set aside to pay for their care. "I crunched the numbers to figure out if we had enough money to care for them until they're 100," Mary said. The answer was "probably not," at least not without the children pitching in.

The cost of LTC comes as a shock to many elders and their families because, unlike hospital care, it is not fully covered by medicare. The rates vary tremendously, anywhere from about $1,800 to $15,000 monthly and up, depending on the type of facility, room and extras.

As with everything in the eldercare field, the nomenclature is unduly complicated and can cause confusion. Long-term-care homes are facilities that provide nursing care and personal care 24/7. They are also sometimes called nursing homes because, traditionally, they were overseen by a nurse. Roughly 190,000 elders are living in government-subsidized long-term-care facilities in Canada, according to the Canadian Institute for Health Information (CIHI). Almost all the residents are elders, but a significant minority, about 10,000, are younger people living with severe disabilities who require around-the-clock assistance.

Then there are retirement homes, assisted living facilities, continuing care homes, lodges, supportive housing and more, where varying levels of care can be provided, but not 24/7 and rarely with nurses on site. There are roughly 170,000 elders living in these facilities. All told, about 350,000 Canadians over 65—about 7 percent of elders—live in these communal settings.

The distinction between long-term-care facilities and retirement homes is an important one, especially from a financial perspective. In long-term-care facilities (known as CHSLDs in Quebec) care is covered as it would be in a hospital. Residents pay only for accommodation (and that cost is regulated) and any extras they want to purchase. In other residential facilities, care is not necessarily covered, so costs can escalate quickly.

Canada also has a strange mix of state-owned (usually by municipalities), not-for-profit and for-profit care homes, roughly in equal numbers. But funding for the care offered in homes comes almost exclusively from the provincial governments, who contract services from the homes.

There is significant political debate about whether for-profit operators should be allowed in the sector. Canada does not have private hospitals, but it does have a lot of private long-term-care homes. Given how care is financed, profits are made by squeezing workers; in recent years there have been significant reductions in the nursing component of care, as well as stagnant (and sometimes falling) wages for PSWs. Private for-profit operators argue that these same trends are seen in not-for-profit and state-owned homes and are a result of underfunding, not profit-taking.

A report by the BC Seniors Advocate found that the province spends $2 billion annually on LTC, of which $1.3 billion is contracted out to 174 care homes. Those payments generated only $37 million in net profits, and they were not evenly distributed, with just eighteen homes making profits in excess of $1 million. In Ontario, by comparison, the three biggest for-profit providers—Extendicare, Sienna Senior Living and Chartwell Retirement Residences—paid out $1.5-billion in dividends to shareholders over the past decade, but that money comes from a mix of long-term care and retirement homes, and the latter are far more profitable. The

BC Advocate also found significant differences in how money is spent: not-for-profit homes spend, on average, $10,000 a year more on direct care of residents; for-profit homes spend significantly more on building expenses. And both for-profit and not-for-profit homes routinely failed to deliver the hours of care they were funded to deliver.

"Every country and every province has great and poor providers," says Dr. Tamara Daly, a political economist and health services researcher at York University in Toronto. "There are fantastic not-for-profits, and great for-profit homes, and there are some in each category who simply shouldn't be operating." But her bottom line is that, like other health institutions funded by the state, such as hospitals, care homes should not be businesses generating profits. "The research is clear on this: there is no doubt that reducing profit-taking would improve care, and we really need to improve care."

The extension of this debate is whether LTC should be considered a "medically necessary" service under the terms of the Canada Health Act. Some activists would like to see the law revised, while others argue that creating parallel legislation such as a Canada Long-Term-Care Act would be a wiser approach. But there is virtually unanimity across the political spectrum and among supporters of not-for-profit and for-profit models alike on one point: the federal government should take a much greater active interest in eldercare, specifically by injecting significant funds into the long-term-care sector. While Ottawa spent more than $300 billion in 2020 on direct relief programs related to Covid-19—everything from wage replacement programs to support for farmers—nothing had been offered to the hard-hit long-term-care sector.

As mentioned above, Anna and Peter Huang now live in the Glebe Centre, a not-for-profit long-term-care facility in downtown Ottawa.

Between them, the couple pays almost \$5,500 a month, which is pretty well the bare minimum for private accommodation. In Ontario, there are three levels of accommodation available:

Basic	\$62.18/day	\$1,891.31 monthly
Semi-private	\$74.96/day	\$2,280.04 monthly
Private	\$88.82/day	\$2,701.61 monthly

Costs are roughly the same in other provinces. Low-income earners can apply for subsidies, but they cover only basic accommodation, and that can sometimes mean living in a ward room with three or four beds.

While \$2,700 a month can sound like a steep rent for a senior, it covers nursing and personal care as well as food, cleaning and other services. The costs paid by residents—about \$32,000 a year each for the Huangs—cover only a fraction of the cost of operating the building and the bed. Governments pay an additional \$80,000 to \$90,000 per resident per year to cover the costs of care—significantly less than it would cost if the residents were in a hospital.

Long-term-care facilities receive the funding in envelopes, on a per diem basis. For example, in Ontario the daily payments are as follows:

Nursing and personal care	\$102.34
Program and support services	\$12.06
Raw food	\$9.54
Other accommodation	\$56.52
TOTAL	\$180.46

That translates to over $5400 per resident monthly. Long-term-care homes get additional funds if they have high-needs patients, or if the facilities are smaller. (They can also have payments clawed back if their beds are not 100 percent full.) Those additional payments are calculated using a complex algorithm that requires workers to do regular detailed assessments. Basically, resources are allocated based on patients' acuity (the severity of illness or disability), but the tools used are imprecise. They tend to favour patients with acute conditions like heart failure. Patients with dementia are not considered acute, so homes with many such patients get less money, which is counterintuitive because their care tends to require a lot more time and staff. To make matters worse, because of staffing problems, assessments are not always done regularly, and the result, paradoxically, is that homes don't get additional funds that would help hire more staff.

In addition to the money for daily provision of care, homes receive a construction subsidy, again on a per diem basis, that ranges from $16.65 to $23.03 for a period of twenty-five years. Rather than make capital investments, governments count on home operators to build facilities and recoup their investments over many years.

While long-term-care and retirement homes are designed for very different populations, the lines are increasingly blurring. Retirement homes and other facilities without around-the-clock nursing and personal care are seeing their residents require increasingly complex care. But, unlike long-term-care homes, they have far more leeway in what they can charge. The quality and costs vary wildly, depending on the luxury of the home and the services purchased. The big difference in retirement homes (which are regulated but not subsidized) is that the care provided is generally purchased separately, and those costs can add up quickly. For example, two hours daily of PSW care purchased from an agency at $35 an hour translates into about $2,000 monthly in additional costs on top of rent that can easily be $3,000.

Because retirement homes are privately run, they have adapted quickly to the changing demographics and offer different levels of care. Independent supported living homes provide a homelike environment with the option to add extra care à la carte, as needed. Assisted living facilities also provide a homelike environment, but care services such as dressing, bathing and grooming are included in the price. There are also retirement homes that offer care specifically for people with mild dementia, such as social, recreational and fitness activities. These "memory care" programs can easily cost $7,000 a month or more. All of these facilities offer everything from basic, apartment-like rooms to premium residences with hotel-style amenities. The retirement home sector is growing much more quickly than LTC because this is where there is money to be made.

Although access to LTC is based on need, even elders with advanced dementia and complex needs can't always get in, and the waits can be long—an average of 100 days for patients waiting in hospital and more than 150 days for those waiting in the community (at home or in a nursing home). In Ontario alone, there are thirty-six thousand people on the wait list for a long-term-care bed.

One of the most common complaints of families is that, when a bed becomes available, they have to decide quickly, within forty-eight to seventy-two hours, whether to accept the placement or not. The lists are managed by local health authorities—in Ontario, the Local Health Integration Network (LHIN)—and operators are penalized if the beds are empty for more than a few days. Refusing a spot can mean going back to the bottom of the list. "They really push hard for you to take the first bed available, to settle for just anything," Mary Huang says. Peter Huang waited sixteen months and Anna Huang eighteen months to end up where they wanted to be.

The Conference Board of Canada estimates that, by 2035, Canada needs to build 199,000 more long-term beds to meet demand among the aging population. That would cost a whopping $64 billion, and that doesn't include operating costs. Yet there is virtual unanimity among the experts that simply building more beds under the current model would solve nothing, and might even exacerbate our problems. "The last thing we need is more beds where the care is not great. What we need is better care," Dr. Sinha says.

The right care at the right place at the right time is a mantra that can't be repeated often enough. The Canadian Institute for Health Information estimates that about one in four people living in long-term-care homes don't need to be there; some experts believe the real number could be as high as one in two.

In Canada, about 80 percent of spending on eldercare goes to institutions and 20 percent to home care. In some European and Nordic countries, that ratio is reversed. There is no single ideal; the choices are ultimately societal and political.

Yet Canada is an outlier amongst developed nations not only for how much it spends on institutional care but also for the types of institutions it operates. The average long-term-care home in this country has about 150 beds, but some have as many as 400. Large homes tend to be located on the outskirts of cities, or even in industrial areas, where land is cheaper. Many long-term-care homes were built in the 1960s and 1970s. Not only are they aging, but they weren't built for the needs of today's patients. For example, the corridors are narrow and there are often stairs, while about 70 percent of long-term-care patients now use wheelchairs and about as many have dementia.

In some parts of the country, there are still ward-style accommodations with three or four beds per room, and they were the hardest hit by the outbreak of coronavirus because infection control is far more difficult in shared spaces. Yet there is a reluctance to eliminate ward rooms because it would mean a loss of about five thousand beds in a system that already has lengthy wait lists, and it would also increase accommodation costs.

The trend worldwide is to build care homes on a much smaller scale and integrate them into the community, with a more homey physical environment. Large care homes have industrial kitchens and/or food services that are contracted out. Meals are served at specific times, often in large dining rooms with thirty-two to sixty-four residents eating at one time. A large cadre of uniformed staff such as janitors and care aides are employed, and there tends to be a lot of turnover. Tasks—everything from bathing to feeding patients—are completed in an assembly line fashion for efficiency's sake.

In smaller homes—and sometimes larger homes broken down into smaller units of ten to twelve residents—the approach is different. Staff wear street clothes, and their shifts are less programmed, allowing workers to be responsive to residents' needs. Meals are prepared on site, sometimes with the participation of residents. There's less staff turnover.

Over the years, a number of alternative models have developed, such as Butterfly Care, Green House and Dementia Village. All of them have peculiarities that distinguish them (and allow them to be commercialized), but they also have a couple of key elements in common. Most importantly, they all embrace relationship-based care rather than the transactional care that is the norm in Canada. The staff-to-resident ratios are excellent, 1:5 or less. Staff have a lot of responsibility but also a lot of power and respect, something that is almost unheard of in Canada's care homes. And crucially, none of these lauded models takes a cookie-cutter approach; they focus on an individual's needs, not on tasks to be completed. The underlying philosophy of all these innovative approaches is basically the same: the person comes first.

"Good care comes down to relationships," says Donna Duncan, CEO of the Ontario Long Term Care Association. But the way LTC is funded and overseen in Canada makes these kinds of approaches almost impossible. "The legislation we have is highly prescriptive and very restrictive. It doesn't allow for much innovation."

Duncan says that funding is also an issue, particularly the amount allocated for staffing, which does not allow for decent ratios. "It's not just about money, though, it's about how we spend the money." Long-term-care operations, whether they are private, public or not-for-profit, don't have any wiggle room. Homes in Ontario receive funding in twenty-two different envelopes; the staffing money can only go to staff, the food money can only go to food, and so on. The result is that budgets are squeezed, and squeezed some more. In addition, while governments talk constantly about providing better care to residents, such as a minimum of four hours daily of direct care, the funding provided barely allows for three hours of care daily. Failure is built into the funding formula.

Ms. Duncan says long-term-care homes have been vilified because of the pandemic. Some of the criticisms are justified, she acknowledges, but overall, homes offer excellent care with the resources they have, and the problems that exist are the result of policies over which individual homes have no control. "What Covid-19 exposed was the overall neglect of seniors in society," she says. As such, the reforms required are broad societal changes, not just more beds, more inspections or more regulations.

"Fixing the eldercare system begins with asking some really basic questions like, 'Who are we serving?', 'How can we make their care safe?' and 'How can we make their lives fulfilling?'" Duncan says.

The difficulty is that there is not much data to answer those fundamental questions. "In long-term care, we have public funding but private data," says Dr. Daly of York University. "I'm a big fan of stats and data, but we don't collect the right kind and we don't use the data we do have properly."

The Royal Society report also bemoaned the dearth of data. The panel said that even the most basic information, like number of long-term-care beds, is inexact, based on estimates. We don't have a good idea why people end up in LTC, whether they need to be there and how long they stay. (There is some provincial data that suggests that, on average, residents live in LTC for less than eighteen months, and virtually all of them die within that short period.)

Dr. Daly says data on the quality of care, quality of work life of staff, and quality of life of residents are all sorely lacking. This is important, she says, because "there is a clear relationship between a good work environment and quality of care." She says there's a need not only for a decent salary and benefits but also to have autonomy and decision-making power.

Dr. Daly says that proper measuring of quality and safety of care is also crucial. For example, one of the key measures of safety in long-term-care homes is falls, but the data is aggregated, not individualized. "If a home records ten falls, we don't know if it's one person falling ten times or ten different people falling. We also don't know the severity—if it's someone falling out of bed or just a couple of inches." What you measure can also create perverse incentives, she notes. To prevent falls, long-term-care homes put people in wheelchairs, but that's bad for their health. It also increases their acuity score (the measure of how sick and disabled they are), which results in the home getting more money—for what is essentially bad care.

Spurred on by the high number of deaths occurring in long-term-care homes during the pandemic, journalists across the country went looking for data on quality of care, as well as oversight and inspections. What they found was not very comforting. Even before coronavirus, outbreaks of infectious disease were routine, everything from influenza to legionnaires' disease. In the US, an estimated 380,000 people in institutional care die of infections annually. Another 90,000 suffer from pressure ulcers. As a general rule, Canadian numbers are about one-tenth of those in the US, which would still make them shockingly large.

CBC News reported that in 2019, only nine of Ontario's 626 long-term-care facilities had undergone "resident quality inspections," the most thorough form of oversight. Four years earlier, virtually every home had undergone this level of inspection. Now inspections are done more on a reactive basis, following complaints. In Quebec, long-term-care homes are inspected only once every three years on average, and the reviews are done between the hours of 9 a.m. and 5 p.m., and not when most problems occur on understaffed overnight shifts. *La Presse* revealed that the province has only seven inspectors for eldercare homes, compared with eighteen inspectors for the well-being of animals. This prompted union president Christian Daigle of the Syndicat de la fonction publique du Québec to say: "We treat animals better than our elders."

CHAPTER 4

Home Sweet Home

Ask anyone where they want to live out the final years of their life and the answer, almost 100 percent of the time, will be "home"—in comfortable, familiar surroundings, with their family, pets, garden, their own food, own bed, own schedule and own rules.

But living at home until the end is a lot more difficult than many people realize, especially into your 80s and 90s. The daily chores and upkeep of the home, from grocery shopping to shovelling the walk, become more difficult, sometimes impossible. Getting around can be a challenge too, especially if you no longer drive. With age, chronic illnesses accumulate, the body becomes more frail, and the mind can be ravaged by dementia. For those who live alone, who are far from family, or whose partner is ailing, the challenges can be redoubled.

Aging in place, however desirable, is easier said than done. Medicare may be a Canadian birthright, with accessible and affordable physician and hospital services available, but home care is another matter altogether. There's no guarantee adequate home care will be available, let alone funded by the public system. The cost can be as much as, or more than, accommodation in a long-term-care home.

Just ask Frank Palmer.

Between the time his wife, Irene, was diagnosed with dementia in 2007 and her death in May 2020, the retired federal civil servant estimates that he spent in excess of $1 million on her care, in addition to what she was afforded in the public system. The bulk of the money went to pay for home care, to ensure she could live and die where she wanted, in her comfortable Toronto home.

"I was determined to keep Irene at home because I wanted her to live in dignity to the end. It required some sacrifices, but she was worth it." But Frank was quick to acknowledge that the choice is only open to people with money. He was a lifelong civil servant and his wife was a registered nurse, so they were comfortable. "We were frugal and we invested our money well," Frank says. They had also benefited from a significant inheritance, all of which made the stay-at-home decision possible. He is the first to admit that pushing people into institutional care is the system's default position and doing otherwise requires a lot of determination and pigheadedness.

"The system sucks—please excuse my language," Frank says. "When it comes to home care, they will give you the bare minimum, and if you're capable of paying anything privately, they will give you even less."

It wasn't supposed to be this way. When medicare was born six decades ago, the idea was to begin by providing universal access to hospital and physician care, because the costs of those services were resulting in some going without care and others being harmed financially, even bankrupted. The next step was to gradually expand public health insurance into other essential areas, including prescription drugs, home care, LTC and dental care. Many developed countries have done just that, but Canada's public health insurance system, medicare, remains frozen in time—this, despite monumental demographic and societal changes that have made home care more essential than ever, and despite countless inquiries and commissions over the years that have called for reform.

In its landmark 2002 report, *Building on Values, the Future of Health Care in Canada*, the Commission on the Future of Health Care in Canada (known colloquially as the Romanow Commission) concluded that expanding access to home care was one of the keys to reforming medicare and building a more robust health system. They labelled home care "the next essential service."

Roy Romanow, a former Saskatchewan premier, and his fellow commissioners noted that during their exhaustive review of the health system there was near-unanimous support for the idea of shifting care out of institutions and into the community and the home. They acknowledged that, given a choice, virtually everyone would opt to live and die at home. The commissioners wrote:

> The advantages are obvious. People get to stay in their own homes with the assurance that someone will be there to monitor their health. For some people, especially seniors and people with disabilities, it means they can maintain their independence. The costs are generally lower than keeping people in hospital . . . [T]here is growing evidence that investing in home care can save money while improving care and the quality of life for people who would otherwise be hospitalized or institutionalized in long-term care facilities.

Yet, despite the strong language in the body of the report, the final recommendation was for an incremental approach. The commissioners said home care should be included as a "medically necessary" service in the Canada Health Act, and therefore publicly funded the way hospital care and physician services are. The commission also called for the creation of a Home Care Transfer in addition to the existing Canada Health Transfer (the mechanism used to transfer federal money to the provinces, which accounts for about 20 percent of overall spending). But the report specified that, to begin with, home care should be covered only for home mental health case management, post-acute medical care, post-acute rehab, and palliative, end-of-life care. This limited provision of home care would cost about $1 billion a year and be considered a floor on which to build. The idea that elders with chronic health issues could be cared for at home rather than in institutions like long-term-care homes was considered a good idea in principle but only to be pursued "as resources permit." In the short term, broader provision of home care services was deemed unrealistic and too expensive. Once again, Canada made the decision to cling to its hospital-centric approach and elders would continue being kicked to the curb or, rather, into institutional care.

Although the Romanow Commission argued that a "strong case can be made for taking the first step in 35 years to expand coverage under the Canada Health Act," politicians did not make that leap. This was no surprise. There is good reason to suppose that doing so would open a Pandora's box of conflicting demands for expansion of coverage. Others worry that if the Canada Health Act is revised, existing protections—such as the ban on user fees—could be eroded.

Still, in the wake of the report, there was immense political pressure to invest more money in the floundering public health system, with or without legislative change. In September 2004, Prime Minister Paul Martin announced a "10-Year Plan to Strengthen Health Care" that included $41 billion in new funding. The injection of cash, touted as the "fix for a generation," was supposed to reduce surgical wait times, bolster primary care, provide catastrophic drug coverage and improve home care. It was a bold political move, and the provinces were eager to get more money, but the gesture wasn't enough to get the federal Liberals re-elected.

The approach was also fundamentally flawed. The funding deal, known as the 2004 Health Accord, was supposed to provide, among other things, "first dollar coverage" for certain home care services. (That terminology, used by insurance plans, means there are no user fees or deductibles.) The funding was also to be directed to home care services that substituted for in-hospital care, for example intravenous medication, wound care, or end-of-life palliative care at home. In other words, it was like giving more money to hospitals, because it allowed them to offload some services onto home care agencies. There was nothing promised to elders with chronic illnesses who wanted to remain in their homes, an area where the needs were greatest.

An even bigger problem with the Health Accord, though, was that the money provided didn't come with any strings attached, or any checks and balances, so there is no way of knowing if it was ever spent on home care. The additional $4 billion a year simply flowed into perpetuating the status quo for another decade.

In 2019, the latest year for which detailed data are available, Canada spent $264 billion on health care, with the bulk of the money going to hospitals ($70.2 billion), prescription drugs ($40.4 billion) and physician services ($39.9 billion), according to the Canadian Institute for Health Information. In the summary of national expenditures that it publishes annually, home care does not have a separate category, principally because services provided and funding sources vary tremendously between jurisdictions. However, in recent years CIHI has done extensive work to measure home care spending and estimates that public spending alone was about $9.2 billion nationwide in 2018. Canadians spent another $5.4 billion purchasing services from privately owned home care agencies in 2017, according to Statistics Canada. But another detailed estimate, by the National Institute on Ageing, found that public home care spending was $4 billion and private spending another $2 billion, for a total of $6 billion. In other words, somewhere between $6 billion and $15 billion a year is spent on home care, but not in any systematic or coordinated manner. The lack of data is telling. To paraphrase the legendary economist John Kenneth Galbraith, in public policy, "if you don't count it, it doesn't count."

While provincially funded home care programs have existed since the 1970s, there has always been tremendous variation between regions in the extent of coverage provided in terms of both hours and cost, as well as significant differences in who provides the service.

Another reason it's difficult to calculate home care spending with any precision is that there is no common definition. The term is generally used to describe an array of services that allows patients with a mental or physical incapacity to remain at home and receive the care they need. That care ranges from professional services such as nursing and physiotherapy to personal care and assistance with activities of daily living, including bathing, toileting and transferring, and also covers homemaking to assist with cleaning, laundry and meal preparation as well as services such as adult day care and Meals on Wheels. Often the goal of home care is to prevent or delay the need for hospital or long-term residential care.

Over time, there has been a growing emphasis on using home care as an extension of the hospital, principally to get surgical patients off the ward more quickly in order to free up beds in overcrowded hospitals. "We've become a post-acute decant—heal the wound and get out," says Sue VanderBent, the CEO of Home Care

Ontario. In that province alone, there are almost 100,000 home care visits a day, but they are designed largely to provide a specific service such as changing a wound dressing or giving a bath in as little as fifteen minutes. "We're doing a lot, and we're doing it on a very thin dime," VanderBent says.

But she is the first to admit that the focus on acute care substitution means that the home care system—which, in fact, is not a system in any way—is not serving the needs of the growing cohort of elders who want to remain at home into their 80s, 90s and 100s. "Home care today is task-oriented: short baths, getting people dressed, some feeding. It's nowhere near comprehensive," VanderBent says. "We're not looking after enough of the people who are getting older and frailer, the people who are clamouring for home care, in the way that we should, because the funding isn't there."

Ontario has a $63.5-billion annual health care budget. Of that total, a little over $3 billion is spent on home care, of which $2 billion is for direct service provision and $1 billion for assessment and navigation. The fact that one-third of the entire budget goes to administration speaks to the bureaucratic nature of home care. A lot of time, energy and money is spent trying to ensure that clients get the strict minimum, in order to stretch resources. Patients, families, health care workers and service providers alike all despair about the rigidity and parsimony.

"We have no funding, no structure, no organization in the sector. Even the government doesn't understand how home care works, or how it should work," VanderBent says.

Ontario is not unique in terms of being overstretched. Coverage varies widely between one province and another. Some provide a monthly dollar amount to individuals, some impose hourly limits, some cap home care spending at the equivalent of what

LTC would cost. The one commonality is that no jurisdiction provides a level of care that could remotely be considered comprehensive, especially for elders who want to live out their days at home. Ontario, for example, will cover a maximum of ninety hours of care every thirty days—essentially, no more than three hours daily, with few exceptions. People often end up in LTC, at much greater cost, for want of a few hours of nursing or homemaking services, all because the home care system is notoriously inflexible and irrational. According to Statistics Canada, more than 900,000 Canadians receive some home care services, but another 430,000 have unmet home care needs.

Home care is also the only publicly funded health service where care is provided based on hard financial caps and arbitrary limits rather than medical need. Imagine if we told a cancer patient: "You need twelve hours of radiation treatment, but—sorry—we have a three-hour limit." Or if we said: "Your public health insurance will cover cancer surgery, but you will have to hire someone privately to sew you back up."

The practical implication is that people who want to keep a loved one at home have to top up the care provided by the state by purchasing supplementary private services. "Family-funded care is common now," VanderBent says. Most home care agencies, both not-for-profit and for-profit, provide home care both for the state and for individuals, often simultaneously. But there is also a burgeoning underground market, where desperate families turn to unlicensed care providers to save a few dollars, and to ensure there is continuity in their care.

Costs can quickly add up, to a staggering level. "If you don't have some dollars in your back pocket, you can't do this," Frank Palmer says. He spent $150,000 on home care services in the last year of his wife's life. Unlike many others, however, he was willing and able to make that investment even though, at the outset, he had no idea how the cost of care would balloon.

Irene Palmer was diagnosed with dementia in 2007, at age 73. She had been showing signs earlier, losing her train of thought and getting lost on a familiar trip downtown on the subway. She and Frank decided to undergo dementia screening together. "She was an RN, so she knew what was going on. The diagnosis was not a big surprise, but it was disappointing because she lost her driver's licence and that really restricted her social activities," Frank says.

As happens with many spouses of someone with dementia, Frank gradually found himself taking over a number of day-to-day functions, such as driving, shopping and cooking. "I didn't think too much of it. It was just something I accepted, that life was changing, as it does when you get older."

When his wife began having trouble feeding and dressing herself, she was allocated one hour of care daily. "But it was never an hour, you were lucky to get thirty minutes. The workers just did the task and wanted to get out of there as quickly as possible." Frank doesn't blame the workers for the abysmal care, but rather a system that runs on cheap labour and piecework. He began supplementing with private providers, most of whom worked in blocks of three hours minimum.

As long as Irene's health was deteriorating gradually, the care load was manageable. However, life changed dramatically in early 2013. The couple were spending the winter in Fort Myers, Florida, when Irene suffered an asthma attack and a fall. "I took her to the hospital. We walked in hand in hand, but she didn't walk out," Frank recalls. Her health declined precipitously, to the point where she ended up in intensive care, and then was transferred to the ICU of a Toronto hospital. "They told us that the prognosis was grim, that she would be going home in a box. But I said: 'No, Irene's going home.'"

At that point, Frank realized some serious home care would be needed. He reached out to the Community Care Access Centre, the Ontario agency that oversaw home care at that time. "It was difficult to even get the basics, so she could be fed and bathed," he says. So he topped up care by purchasing services from private providers. His biggest frustration was not the cost but the lack of organization. There were endless assessments, care plans, and a constant churn of workers. Worse yet, none of the agencies spoke to each other, shared information or coordinated care. "It drove me crazy. I ended up hiring a consultant who, after considerable effort, got all the parties at the table and managed to come up with a single care plan for Irene."

Frank says he took a businesslike approach to his wife's illness. "The way I approached it was: I'm the CEO of the house and the primary role of everyone who comes into the house is to look after Irene, to make sure she has the best quality of life possible." At times, he could have up to seven workers in the house in a single day.

Of course, there was pressure to move Irene to a long-term-care facility. Even at $10,000 monthly for a private room, the expense would be less, not to mention all the effort required to coordinate care and the personal caregiving. Frank did visit at least fifteen different homes in the Toronto area, but despite the cost, and the all-consuming nature of caring for a dementia patient, he always came to the same conclusion: there's no place like home.

"One thing I knew in my heart is that Irene enjoyed being at home, in her home. We always made sure she was engaged in home life. She would help in the kitchen. She had a chair, her favourite chair, where she would sit and watch the birds at the bird feeder and smile," Frank says. "I just didn't see that happening in a long-term-care home. I visited a lot of them and one thing I didn't see was a lot of smiles."

With advanced dementia, the maximum time Irene was allocated was three hours daily. That was topped up with four hours daily of private care. In the final weeks, when his wife was receiving palliative care, there was health care staff caring for her from 7:30 a.m. to 10 p.m., and then Frank would do the overnight shift alone.

On May 2, 2020, more than thirteen years after her home care odyssey began, Irene Palmer died in her bed, in her home, as per her wishes, with her husband of forty-three years by her side.

When asked if he has any regrets, Frank pauses and reflects. "Every once in a while, you have a little twinge, wishing maybe you have done more things, had more of the normal life of a retiree. But to ensure the respect and dignity of someone I loved, no sir, I don't regret it at all."

What he does regret, rue even, is that so little is done to make home care a viable option for all.

Shirlee Sharkey is president and CEO of SE Health, one of Canada's oldest and largest home care agencies, with 6.5 million home care visits a year. St. Elizz, as it is known colloquially, has been around since 1908 and has changed dramatically over that period, always positioning itself as an innovator. Sharkey is a thoughtful critic of the way care, and particularly home care, is delivered in Canada. She says the Covid-19 crisis exposed many problems in long-term-care homes, but she really wants politicians and policy-makers to retain two related lessons: "Home is a safe place to be. And home is where people want to be."

Sharkey is particularly frustrated by the fact that everyone wants to age in place in their home, but so few actually have that choice. Deciding where to live out your final years should be the norm, not the exception, she says, pointing out that the Palmers' experience highlights virtually everything that is wrong with home care, for clients, families, health professionals, care delivery organizations and governments.

She says families are invariably unsatisfied with their home care experience because they have to deal with multiple providers who give uncoordinated care that focuses on completing specific tasks within a set time limit. Home care clients are allocated blocks of care, but not necessarily the care they want or need. "Bureaucracy has gone nuts in our sector," Sharkey says. "For example, families complain that we don't have care plans. But we do. The problem is, we have ten of them—one by the nurse, one by the coordinator, one by the PSW, one by the supervisor, and so on—and none of them are customized to a person's needs."

If there is no strong-willed, dedicated family member to navigate the complicated bureaucracy, elders often end up in institutional care by default, and that is especially true of those who live alone.

The task-oriented nature of home care frustrates health workers as much as it does families. So does the workload. Kim Clunas, a veteran PSW based in London, Ontario, says that workers are so rushed to complete their duties that there is little or no time to interact with patients, which is an essential part of providing good care. "I've had as many as twenty-two clients in eight hours. You can't treat people properly like that, it's just chaos." Families often complain that workers are late or don't show, and they are right to be angry, Clunas says. But they also have to realize that, in addition to seeing patients, PSWs have to arrange appointments and travel between clients' homes, often in an unreasonably tight time frame.

"My job as a PSW is to make people feel good and look good. You always wish you could do more, but you have to be okay with doing your best in the time you have," she explains. Despite the challenges, Clunas says the work is rewarding, particularly when clients appreciate the seemingly simple things. For example, bathing a patient is not simply about cleaning the person's body; it's also a good time to do an assessment of the client's physical and mental state, and an opportunity for intimate conversations, where people can express their expectations and fears. Better yet, a well-trained PSW can help clients learn to bathe themselves again, an approach called re-enabling. Sadly, those intangibles are not appreciated or rewarded in a system that values checking off items on lists instead of satisfying clients. Clunas, who has worked in four different provinces, says the issues are the same all over the country. Everyone is trying to cut corners to save a bit of money, and it takes a toll on both workers and family members.

After almost thirty years in the field, she decided that, instead of being an employee, she would start her own one-person agency. There are no more fifteen-minute visits for her. Instead, she does longer, three-hour stints, and sometimes even overnight care. More importantly, Clunas gets to know her clients as people. "If you have the right rapport, the right connection, the clients feel like family," she says. "Then it's like, 'Wow, this is why I do this work.'"

Shirlee Sharkey, who worked for many years as a home care nurse before becoming an administrator, says care delivery agencies get blamed for the poor state of home care, and workers often see them as the bad guys, but government regulations and limited funding mean "we are unable to deliver on our mission." Health care is a hands-on business, so staffing is the most essential component. Yet home care agencies in particular have trouble attracting and retaining staff, for a variety of practical reasons. Workers such as nurses and PSWs get paid significantly less in the home care sector than in long-term-care homes or hospitals, often $5 to $7 per hour less, even if they do the same work. The wage disparity is exacerbated by the fact that workers are often paid for 15-, 30- or 60-minute blocks, and not for their travel time between clients. After the Covid-19 debacle in long-term-care homes, governments vowed to hire more workers and pay them better, but that action has the effect of making the staffing problem even more acute in the home care sector.

At the systems level, health authorities and provincial governments are faced with their own challenges, namely the demand for and cost of services growing exponentially as the population ages and as baby boomers become increasingly vocal about wanting choice in where their care is provided. At the same time, other parts of the health system—hospitals, primary care, LTC and more—are also clamouring for more funding, all against the backdrop of a shrinking tax base. Because home care is a relatively small sector, and one with few powerful voices, it is left to languish on the back burner.

Sharkey says there are indeed many challenges, but the answer is not to try to fix home care in a vacuum. "If you ask me, the whole system needs to be turned on its head. We need to design care around where people live, not around institutions." She believes it's also essential to create a fulfilling work environment, to empower health professionals to deliver care in a smart, responsive manner.

The typical response to these calls for reform is almost always the same. As the Romanow Commission report put it two decades ago, the argument is always that making it the norm to age at home is a great idea, but making that fundamental shift overnight is too expensive, so it has to be done gradually.

Sharkey thinks that's nonsense. In her view, most care can be delivered efficiently and cost-effectively in the home, and that position is backed up by some heavyweight research, including the *National Evaluation of the Cost-Effectiveness of Home Care*, by Marcus Hollander and Neena Chappell of the University of Victoria. This report concluded that investing smartly in home care would save money while improving care and the quality of life of patients.

"There's enough money in the system, it's just all over the damn place, and we don't get value for money," Sharkey says. The starting point for reforming home care, she insists, should not be about the cost but about values. "We need a large societal discussion about how to treat the aging population. How can we ensure that everyone controls their destiny? There's no perfect answer to that question, but we do know that what we have now is inadequate, and it needs a fundamental rethink."

Gail Donner, who headed an Ontario review of home care that produced the 2015 report *Bringing Care Home*, reached a similar conclusion: "Not everyone agrees on the solutions, but no one thinks the status quo is acceptable." The Donner report said the overarching goal should be to provide all elders with the "right care at the right time in the right place." That is not happening because there is no coordinated strategy, wide variability in eligibility and access, and little or no accountability for outcomes.

In its recommendations, the Donner Commission said that, before they make any decisions, Ontario's elders and their families should have a clear understanding of what services they can expect under what circumstances. Right now, that's a guessing game because there is no defined "basket of services" covered by publicly funded insurance, and no coordination between health and social services. The critique, though made of Ontario, applies to every province. The Donner report also strongly endorsed self-directed funding—essentially, allocating a fixed amount of money to a patient/family and allowing them to purchase the services they feel are most appropriate. The commission's final recommendation, that someone be appointed to ensure the recommendations would be implemented, was not acted on—and so, like many other well-considered reports, it was left to gather dust.

Just how neglected the home care sector is became glaringly obvious during the Covid-19 pandemic. In a bid to ensure hospitals would not be overwhelmed by pandemic patients, they were emptied of all but the most gravely ill. Nursing homes and long-term-care homes, already overwhelmed, had to deal with the influx. What got less attention was that most home care clients had their services reduced or suspended altogether, in order to reduce the likelihood that home care clients would contract coronavirus from peripatetic workers. While well-intentioned, the move had grave unintended consequences: Home care workers lost their income and left the sector in droves. Numerous patients, unable to get the care they needed at home, ended up in hospital or in residential care, which is more costly and increased their likelihood of getting infected.

The irony was not lost on leaders in the home care sector: while millions of Canadians were being told to stay safe at home, to shelter in place, some of the most vulnerable in society were being forced out of their homes.

CHAPTER 5

Forgotten: Caring for Elders with Dementia

A thief, kidnapper, slow-motion murderer, Alzheimer's pur-
portedly robs, steals and erases one's memory, mind, personality—even one's very self. That persons with dementia are so
readily envisioned as vanished or vanishing, succumbing to
an especially terrifying, slow-moving, unstoppable vortex of
suffering, surely speaks to anxieties beyond the ordinary fears
of death and disease.

LYNN CASTEEL HARPER
Author, *On Vanishing: Mortality, Dementia, and What It Means to Disappear*

At age 73, John Poole was still hard at work, not interested in retirement or slowing down. For many years he owned a successful
small business in Calgary, but he had sold it and was now working
part-time as a consultant and insurance agent. He also kept very
active—as he had been his whole life—playing hockey, squash and
tennis, running, and more.

But John started to become forgetful and withdrawn. He found
himself sitting for hours staring out the window. He went to his

family doctor but was told that forgetfulness and slowing down are a normal part of getting older.

However, while the risk of dementia does increase with age, it's actually not a normal part of aging.

"We learned later that the doctor knew he had dementia but thought he was doing my dad a favour by not telling him, that it would just cause him to worry," remembers his daughter, Lisa Poole. It would be almost a year before the official diagnosis of vascular dementia, but there was plenty of worry along the way as John's symptoms grew worse.

There is a widespread attitude, even among some medical professionals, that not much can be done about dementia and so a diagnosis is not necessarily helpful. That's not true, of course. Ethical considerations aside, early diagnosis allows for patients and their families to plan for living with their condition, to adapt and possibly even to do rehab.

"It didn't help that we were the poster child for a family that was clueless. We knew absolutely nothing about dementia," Lisa says. That would soon change.

The steep learning curve that comes with a dementia diagnosis is one that many families experience. An estimated 564,000 Canadians are living with dementia, and that number is growing by at least 25,000 a year, according to the Alzheimer Society of Canada. By 2031, the total figure is expected to rise to 937,000. Behind those statistics are individuals—each one a person who will require varying degrees of care—and families who will have some unimaginable challenges thrust upon them.

Dementia is a global pandemic, not one unique to Western countries. Worldwide, about 50 million people have dementia, and there are nearly 10 million new cases annually. For the growing legion of elders, regardless of where they live in the world, there are few things more terrifying than a dementia diagnosis. Like John, people are often left with the impression, reinforced by stereotypes ingrained in popular culture, that loss of memory and loss of control over daily life are inevitable. Yet there are many lifestyle and socio-economic factors that contribute to cognitive decline, and addressing them could reduce the burden of dementia by almost half.

The reality, too, is that while fear of dementia is common, only about 6 to 8 percent of those over 65 are living with dementia at any given time. Mind you, the risk increases sharply with age: about 1 percent of those between 65 and 69 have dementia, but after age 85 it's more than 25 percent. But symptoms and severity vary greatly, as do coping mechanisms.

Dementia is the umbrella term for as many as a hundred different forms of age-related cognitive decline, each with a different constellation of symptoms. By far the best-known form of dementia is Alzheimer disease, which accounts for more than half of all cases. It is thought to be caused by the abnormal buildup of two kinds of protein. One of the proteins is called amyloid, and its deposits form plaques around brain cells; the other protein is called tau, and its deposits form tangles within brain cells. Other types of dementia include vascular dementia, where the brain is damaged by small mini-strokes, known formally as transient ischemic attacks, or damage to blood vessels; Lewy body dementia, caused by the buildup of the protein alpha-synuclein in the parts of the brain that control memory and movement; and frontotemporal dementia (FTD), where proteins build up in the frontal and temporal lobes. Dementia can even be caused by infectious diseases like Creutzfeldt–Jakob disease, also known as mad cow disease. Distinguishing between the various forms is difficult and can usually be confirmed only by a post-mortem examination of the brain.

Regardless of its precise form, dementia is one of the major causes of disability and dependency among elders worldwide. It is also deadly. Officially, more than 8,000 Canadians die annually of dementia, the eighth leading cause of death in Canada. But death certificates greatly underrepresent Alzheimer's and other dementias because, as the condition advances, patients tend to die of infections and heart problems. Based on US research, the real number of deaths is probably in the range of 16,000 to 20,000. While people can live a long time with dementia, almost half of those affected die within five years of diagnosis, a higher mortality rate than most forms of cancer.

The most common early symptom of dementia is declining memory, especially short-term memory. Over time, people can experience difficulty performing familiar tasks, problems with language, disorientation in time and place, poor or decreased judgment, changes in mood or behaviour, withdrawal from social interactions, and, in some cases, paranoia and hallucinations.

Dementia can be overwhelming, not only for the people who have the condition but for their caregivers and families. John Poole's spouse and adult children decided they would care for him on their own at home. That choice is actually the norm; contrary to common perceptions, more than half of people with dementia live at home. For John's family, they managed on their own for a while. But he started to need help with activities of daily living, at which point they hired workers to come into the home. That help can be hard to come by, especially from the publicly funded health system, and the cost of privately purchased care can be steep.

"I know home care is a great idea in theory, but for us it was a complete disaster," Lisa Poole says. She talks of how workers often showed up late—if at all, the turnover in staff was constant, and care aides didn't seem to have any specialized training for dealing with patients with dementia. For example, patients may be unaware of their condition and confused by the presence of strangers, so they will be unco-operative or tell care aides to leave. If a worker doesn't know how to handle that common scenario, a patient may miss out on being fed a meal or getting a bath that day.

Exacerbating the problem for the Pooles was the fact that adult day care programs were hard to come by and those that were available took place in long-term-care homes. "When you're in the early stages of dementia, the last thing you want to do is spend time in one of those facilities. It's a frightening glimpse of your future—a bit like taking a kindergarten kid to a high-security prison," says Lisa.

For John Poole's family, the practical result of unreliable home care and unavailable respite care was that his wife wasn't able to get a break from the daily demands of caregiving, even with the help of her adult children. Caring for a person with dementia, even in the relatively early stages, can be a 24/7 job, especially if they start wandering at night, so respite for caregivers is essential.

Within a year of his diagnosis, it became too difficult to care for John at home, so the family applied for a spot in a long-term-care home. An opening came up relatively quickly, at a home that was privately owned but publicly funded. But the sudden availability turned out to be more of a stressor than a relief. John had lived in the same home for forty-four years, so uprooting him, especially when doctors kept saying stability was important to his health, was not a decision to be taken lightly.

"There was tremendous pressure to make this life-changing decision immediately," Lisa says. The family had twenty-four hours to accept the placement or go back to the bottom of the pile. With tens of thousands of people on the wait lists—thirty-five thousand in Ontario alone—few people dare decline, even if they've never seen the care home or it is hundreds of kilometres away. The Pooles took the spot.

When John arrived, there was no orientation, no slow transition; from one day to the next, he left his long-time family home for a strange new setting. This sudden change would be off-putting for anyone, but was even more so for a dementia patient.

"My father was totally disoriented. He wasn't someone who wandered, but he started waking up at night and walking the halls," Lisa says. Worse yet, even though he was in a "memory ward," where patients are locked in for their safety, when John refused to return to his room, staff would call 911. He was a strapping six foot two, and the lone staff member, usually a tiny woman, could feel intimidated and frightened even though he was not aggressive, just uncooperative. When police or paramedics arrived, they would take John to the hospital, where he would spend hours before getting a cursory once-over and be discharged after a family member came to get him. Such transfers to hospital, when patients are disruptive or sick, are commonplace. One study estimated that 75 percent would be avoidable with proper staffing.

For John, middle-of-the-night visits to Calgary's South Campus Hospital became routine, happening once every couple of weeks. One night he urinated on the floor of the care home—behaviour that is not unusual or unexpected for someone with dementia. The care home decided that he was too difficult to care for and would not be welcome to return. This too is common; understaffed care homes routinely try to send high-needs patients to more specialized facilities.

So, after about eight months in LTC, the hospital became John's new home.

Across Canada, there are more than 7,500 people living in hospitals as they wait for placement in a care home. They are known as "alternate level of care" (ALC) patients, an Orwellian term of the highest order because the care they get is not so much "alternate" as non-existent. In some provinces, like Nova Scotia, fully one-third of beds are filled by ALC patients, the majority of them living with dementia.

The advantage of hospitals is that they have more and better-trained staff, nurses instead of care aides and orderlies. But hospitals have no programming or recreational activities. They are not designed for daily living, so patients like John Poole end up just lying in bed. While Canadian hospitals are perpetually overcrowded, they like (or at least tolerate) ALC patients because they don't really need medical care. Since they get help with activities of daily living like feeding and toileting from orderlies (or, often, family visitors), their presence takes pressure off overworked staff. And if they wander about too much, they are restrained, physically or chemically.

Both chemical restraint (prescribing antipsychotics to patients to sedate them, even though they do not have psychosis) and physical restraint (wheelchair lap belts, bed rails and limb restraints) are frequently used not just in hospitals but also in long-term-care homes. According to the Canadian Institute for Health Information, about one-third of dementia patients are prescribed antipsychotics inappropriately, and that number was much higher just a few years ago. About one in ten dementia patients is also physically restrained daily, although that rate is much lower today than in the past, due to advocacy and lawsuits by families.

On their regular visits to the Calgary South hospital, members of the Poole family drove past a long-term-care facility. Desperate to get their father out of hospital, one day they stopped for a visit to check the place out. They were impressed enough to make the decision to move John again.

"It was a really fancy place, not something my dad would go for, honestly, but we figured the care would be much better," Lisa says. "I'm also embarrassed to say it cost $15,000 a month."

Even more shocking than the price tag was that, despite the luxurious surroundings, the care ended up being the same as in the public facility John had left months earlier. Not only that, but the same people who worked in the public home worked in the private home. "Despite the price, the home was understaffed, the staff lacked proper training, and they didn't really understand dementia."

The family set out to find something better and more affordable, but the search took almost a year. Lisa was extremely frustrated at how difficult it was to get basic information on care homes, and she was determined to address the problem. With the support of the Alzheimer Society of Calgary and the nursing faculty at the University of Calgary, she created a magazine called *Dementia Connections*, which provides information and resources for families with a loved one with dementia.

According to Lisa Poole, one of the most exhausting and frustrating things for families is trying to navigate the complexity of the health and social services systems, especially when they are reeling from a loved one being diagnosed with dementia. "What's really needed is a single point of contact, a person who can actually coordinate care, to help you get home care, long-term care or whatever you need. Families shouldn't have to be doing this on their own," she says.

John Poole's next stop was a small facility close to his old family home. It was as if the family's prayers had been answered. The family loved the location and the look; it was a homelike setting in a residential area, not institutional at all. Staff wore street clothes, not uniforms. They would make home-cooked meals (with residents helping sometimes), and eat with and have tea with their charges. They spent time socializing rather than just carrying out tasks on a rigid schedule. "When it was good, it was outstanding," Lisa says. It was also quite expensive.

The philosophy was to recognize the individuality of each resident, to honour their autonomy, choice, privacy and dignity—in short, to get away from the medical model of care. There are many models out there espousing holistic, person-centred approaches, including the Butterfly model, the Eden Alternative, Green House, Wellspring and the Gentle Care System.

Unfortunately, the situation gave John only eighteen months of stability. "It didn't last," Lisa says. "They were well-intentioned, maybe a bit idealistic, and really in over their heads. They didn't really think out the business model." When the home closed, residents were evicted with just twenty-four hours' notice.

An emergency placement saw John back in the public system, with similar frustrations to his first experience. The home was chronically understaffed and made it clear that it couldn't really meet the needs of people with advanced dementia, especially someone as active as John. "We got him out of there as fast as we could," Lisa recalls.

Along the way, the family became disenchanted with LTC and its limitations. "My biggest regret is that we didn't keep Dad at home longer. With the knowledge we have now, we could have done it, but the system is so cumbersome that it continually pushes people to a higher level of care than they need. It pushes them to institutional care at every turn," Lisa says. The stats bear that out: five years after diagnosis, only one in four people with dementia are still living in the community.

At one point, they considered self-managed care, an approach where families are allocated a fixed amount of money and they can spend it as they see fit to care for their loved one—hiring home care workers, purchasing respite care and so on. The approach is popular with families of children with severe disabilities but is also sometimes used for eldercare. Lisa was excited at the prospect of having more control over her father's care, but she quickly became disillusioned. "Self-managed care is a good idea in theory but not in practice." She attended an information session with her mother and a roomful of people in their 70s and 80s, many of whose first language was not English, and they were subjected to an "advanced income tax seminar coupled with a lot of threats about what would happen if you didn't do things exactly according to the rules." Lisa says it was all too typical of how the health system treats families. "People are already in the worst place of their lives, beaten down, desperate and exhausted, and instead of [being given] relief, they are beaten down some more," she says.

So, in October 2018, John ended up in yet another long-term-care home, his fifth. It was another privately operated, publicly funded home, located in a converted convent. But, like almost all publicly funded LTC in Canada, it was not without added costs. John's family paid extra for a private room and also supplemented his care with a daily visit from a licensed practical nurse (LPN), which is an unspoken necessity given staff shortages.

John's illness had progressed to the point where he used a wheelchair, yet the physical space was not designed for someone with mobility issues. He also had aphasia, an inability to speak, which made the lockdown during Covid-19 particularly frustrating, because family members were essentially unable to communicate with him for months. When a person communicates using facial gestures and touch, all the personal care and medical care in the world is not a substitute for face-to-face contact.

———

John Poole's seven-year journey since his diagnosis has included some time at home, without and with home care, time in hospital as an ALC patient, and stays in multiple care homes, private and public, affordable and unaffordable.

"Five homes in five years is awful, especially for someone with dementia. But what's really awful is that it isn't at all unusual. It's almost the norm," Lisa says.

The other shockingly normal part of the family's experience is the financial cost they have borne. "A lot of Canadians think, because we have medicare and old-age pensions, that once you turn 65, the government will magically take care of you, that they will pay for everything. A lot of people get a big, nasty surprise." After seven years, she explains, "we're cleaned out and we're certainly not alone."

Lisa Poole speaks with authority because, as she grew more informed and engaged as a caregiver, she also became an advocate and activist, and co-chair of the group Dementia Advocacy Canada (DAC). Groups like the Alzheimer Society of Canada provide information and services to patients and families, but because they are charitable organizations that raise money, they have legal and practical limitations on how much they can speak out. DAC believes that people with dementia and their caregivers need to have an unfettered voice in demanding better care. One of the guiding principles of the group is that people with dementia should, whenever possible, speak for themselves. The other co-chair of the group is Mary Beth Wighton of Southampton, Ontario.

Mary Beth had been working as an executive recruiter and corporate trainer, travelling the world and responsible for a global team of IT specialists, but she started making mistakes with routine tasks and found her personality changing. The normally easygoing Mary Beth became "short-fused" with people and had angry outbursts. Her work suffered as she started having trouble remembering data and numbers, and at home she made some terrible investment decisions that cost her dearly.

To figure out what was wrong, Mary Beth visited a gamut of health professionals—therapists, psychologists, psychiatrists and family physicians—where she received a dozen different diagnoses, ranging from hypochondria to depression. "Everyone noted that I had symptoms of dementia, but they all kept saying I was too young to have dementia," she says. So even though she was only 45, she made an appointment with a geriatrician. After a battery of tests, Mary Beth was diagnosed with frontotemporal dementia in September 2012.

Her partner, Dawn Baxter, who had accompanied her to the appointment, said, "Great, we finally know what's wrong. How do we fix it?" The doctor replied bluntly that there was no treatment and no cure, and that Mary Beth should go home and get her affairs in order because she faced inexorable mental decline and would likely be dead within six to eight years. He also said that her driver's licence would be invalidated, effective immediately. "He didn't have the best bedside manner," Dawn comments dryly.

There are few things more devastating than a dementia diagnosis. At age 45, and with the news being delivered without an iota of compassion, it was even more shocking. Many people withdraw and hide because, when you're told your brain is betraying you, the loss feels immediate and profound. Mary Beth was no exception. "The only thing I was prescribed was disengagement: 'Go home and die,'" she says. The depression she had already been experiencing became even more profound.

Gradually, Mary Beth was able to start crawling out of her black hole. Some of her professional training kicked in. Armed with a diagnosis, she realized, she could now get educated about FTD and make a plan. "I thought, 'I'm 45 years old and I have a lot of living left in me,'" she explains. "I decided, 'Well, this is a disease and I'm going to fight it like any other disease I might have gotten, like cancer.'"

Mary Beth's saving grace was connecting with the Murray Alzheimer Research and Education Program (MAREP) at the University of Waterloo. It has an "authentic partnership" approach to working with people living with dementia, family care partners and professionals. "They believe in working with, not for, people with dementia," she says. "They promote engagement, not disengagement." MAREP has four guiding principles: 1) People with dementia have the right to be, and must be, involved in dementia care; 2) Understanding the experiences of dementia from the perspective of those living with dementia is critical to quality of life; 3) People with dementia can continue to grow and learn but need adequate information, resources and support to do so; and 4) Good dementia care requires strong partnerships between all persons involved.

"They told me, 'You know best what you can do.' They said, 'You're young, you're smart, and you can do a lot of things.' And they were right." Mary Beth began doing advocacy work, focused specifically on the view that people with dementia should have a voice and should have rights like everyone else.

Meanwhile, she was working on her own future care plan. She and Dawn visited several long-term-care homes, and the experience only made Mary Beth more determined to remain at home. "Dementia is the only disease where people are still locked up. Why isn't the public outraged that thousands of people—their mothers, their grandmothers—are in locked wards, deprived of their dignity and their liberty?" She rejects out of hand the argument that this sort of confinement is designed to protect people, saying that is the excuse that was used for centuries to lock people away in institutions because they were poor or had physical or developmental disabilities or psychiatric illnesses. "It's not a crime to be sick. If people want to wander, don't imprison them, provide them with a safe place to walk," she insists.

In other words, autonomy and dignity are just as important as medical care and help with activities of daily living. That concept is reflected in Canada's first-ever dementia strategy. On June 17, 2019, the Government of Canada released *A Dementia Strategy for Canada: Together We Aspire*, which has three key objectives: 1) prevent dementia; 2) advance therapies and find a cure; and 3) improve the quality of life of people living with dementia and their caregivers. Ottawa allocated $50 million over five years to kick-start the initiative.

Dr. Saskia Sivananthan, chief research and knowledge translation officer at the Alzheimer Society of Canada, says it is an important document and long overdue. "It has good bones, a lot of good elements, but now we have to act on it." Specifically, she says that to bring the promises to life, there needs to be a detailed implementation strategy, including clear targets and money to implement the changes. The only concrete target in the strategy is that at least 1 percent of all spending should go to research. Dementia care costs about $10.4 billion annually in Canada, which would translate into $104 million for research. Current research spending is $41 million.

Dr. Sivananthan states that the emphasis on prevention is also important for reducing the economic and societal burden of dementia. In a study published in the *Lancet* in July 2020, a blue-ribbon panel of scientists estimated that about 40 percent of dementia cases could be delayed or prevented by implementing a series of lifestyle and public policy changes. The panel, led by

Professor Gill Livingston of University College London, identified several "modifiable risk factors" from childhood through to old age:

- Aim to maintain systolic blood pressure of 130 mm Hg or less in mid-life from around age 40.
- Encourage use of hearing aids for hearing loss and reduce hearing loss by protecting ears from high noise levels.
- Reduce exposure to air pollution.
- Prevent head injury (particularly by targeting high-risk occupations and transport).
- Prevent alcohol misuse and limit drinking to less than twenty-one units per week.
- Stop smoking uptake and support individuals to stop smoking (which the authors stress is beneficial at any age).
- Provide all children with primary and secondary education.
- Lead an active life into mid- and possibly later life.
- Reduce obesity and diabetes.

While there is a lot of grandiose talk about curing dementia—for example, at a 2013 Dementia Summit the leaders of the G8 countries pledged to find a cure by 2025—the reality is that there really are no effective treatments and in recent years many promising drug trials have flopped.

Dr. Sivananthan says that's a stark reminder that we can't suddenly start thinking about dementia only when someone starts needing care; prevention measures need to begin in childhood and continue across the life course. And when people do develop symptoms, we have to focus on their quality of life but also ensure they get rehab to slow the progression of the illness. They also need to be housed appropriately.

"No one is ever excited by the prospect of moving into long-term care because, as it exists, it doesn't meet anyone's needs," Dr. Sivananthan concludes. "Care in the community is where we have to put our emphasis. People with dementia are like everyone else—they want to live at home, in the community, and they want to have the best quality of life possible.

"If we get care right for people with dementia, we get it right for everyone."

CHAPTER 6

Healing Hands

Health care is a hands-on business, and nowhere is that more evident than when it comes to the care of elders. As people age and lose their mobility, dexterity, continence and memory, they depend increasingly on a helping hand from others to assist with essential activities of daily living. Family members play a key role, but so do paid care providers. Many elders' survival relies, day in and day out, on those who feed, bathe, dress and medicate them.

Personal care workers are ubiquitous in the health system: in long-term-care homes, group homes, nursing homes, home care, correctional facilities, hospitals and more. But the profession (or, as some prefer, occupation) is largely unregulated, so it's not even clear how many workers there are nationwide; the best guess is somewhere between 350,000 and 400,000. Even the terms used to describe these workers vary tremendously around the country: care aides, personal support workers (PSWs), continuing care assistants, home support workers, and, in Quebec, *préposés aux bénéficiaires*/orderlies.

Regardless of the nomenclature, the workers who help care for people who are ill or elderly or who need help with daily tasks are racialized women, for the most part. One study found that 90 percent of care workers are women, three-fifths have English or French as a second language (a proxy for being immigrants or refugees) and two-thirds are over the age of 40. These hard-working women are paid lowly wages for back-breaking work, and are largely taken for granted both by the individuals they serve and by the institutions that employ them, as well as by a society whose policies and values have made this work a cornerstone of eldercare.

Josephine Marquez is a care aide in Vancouver with more than twenty-two years' experience. She came to Canada from the Philippines in 1993 to work as a nanny through the Live-In Caregiver Program, which allows immigrants to get work experience and apply for permanent residency, then citizenship. The jump from nanny to care aide is a common trajectory because it requires little training, and the work is plentiful, albeit poorly paid.

"I like helping people," she says when asked why she has stayed so long in an occupation that has a notoriously high turnover rate. About one-third of care aides leave in any given year; many of them take jobs in fast-food restaurants because the pay and hours are better. Only one-third last more than five years; but most of that group, like Marquez, are "lifers" who see the job as a calling.

As much as she loves working with elders, helping the people in her charge has become increasingly difficult and demanding over the past two decades. Not only does she have to care for more patients, but over the years they have become markedly sicker and frailer. Almost 80 percent of long-term-care residents suffer from cognitive decline, up to and including dementia; almost as many have a constellation of other conditions such as diabetes, arthritis, heart failure, COPD and depression. Twenty years ago a number of Marquez's patients could still dress, bathe and feed themselves, but now virtually everyone needs help with each of those multiple-times-a-day tasks.

"When I started, I took care of twelve people during an eight-hour shift, and not all of them needed help all the time," Marquez says. Now, many employers, particularly in private care homes, have split shifts, morning and night, four hours each, where the care aide is responsible for at least eight patients. In other words, the work is more intense and there is no downtime. "Just work, work, work."

The greatest frustration for patients and caregivers alike is how task-oriented and impersonal care provision has become. Specific tasks must be completed within a set time period, like working on the factory floor. There is no time to talk to patients, or to sit and have a cup of tea. "We're always understaffed and we're always busy. It's really not fair to the seniors. When you have to look after too many, they don't get good care. It makes me feel really bad," Marquez says.

The work is physically demanding, too. A petite woman like Marquez lifts people from beds, chairs, wheelchairs and toilets, and sometimes off the floor, dozens of times a day, and they don't (and sometimes can't) always co-operate. "To transport people who are frail, who have dementia, you have to be strong and delicate at the same time," she says. Mechanical aids like lifts can also be used, but they are not always available, and using them is time-consuming. In all her time as a care aide Marquez has never had a severe back injury, which is unusual for someone in her line of work. Almost 15 percent of PSWs suffer workplace injuries annually—a six-times-higher incidence than for firefighters and police officers.

Being a care worker means having to endure being hit, groped, spat on, verbally abused and more. Patients with advanced dementia, in particular, can be disinhibited, confused, frightened or hallucinating, and so they can lash out, a problem that is exacerbated because workers are rushed. "Sometimes they hit you. Sometimes they say things that aren't very nice. The bad words? Oh, yes,"

Marquez says with a laugh. "I just remind myself that they're sick and they don't know what they're doing. I know they're really nice people, so I try to be nice too."

The work can also take a toll on workers' mental health. They witness patients suffering every day, from illnesses and from isolation. Death comes with the territory. In an average 200-bed home, there will be a handful of deaths every month. During the pandemic in the early months of 2020, those numbers soared. Several long-term-care homes had death rates around 40 percent. Marquez says she was lucky to work in a home that did not have an outbreak, but the stress and worry about bringing the coronavirus into a facility was constant. "It was scary. Nobody wants to hurt their patients," she says.

One of the silver linings of the deadly outbreak of Covid-19 in long-term-care homes is that it helped expose the working conditions of care workers, and sparked a debate about staff shortages and pay, and even some action. What is frustrating for workers, though, is that these problems have existed for years, and sometimes decades, and it was common knowledge among everyone from front-line workers to academics that these beleaguered institutions would be hammered by any new infectious disease threat. Some provinces, including Ontario and Quebec, gave some front-line care providers wage increases of $4 per hour during the first wave of the pandemic. However, those raises were rescinded after a few months when it was deemed that the immediate crisis had passed. But the public discussions of how little care workers get paid today tell only part of the story.

Josephine Marquez says she makes about the same wage today as she did two decades ago, although her payment history has been far from static. Until the early 2000s, BC had a master agreement, negotiated provincially, that ensured all workers received the same basic wage and benefits. But the Liberal government changed the legislation, allowing private operators to opt out, and that resulted in widespread contracting out and significant cuts in wages and benefits.

In 2004, Marquez was making $22 an hour and had benefits such as paid holidays and sick days. But then the owners of the home where she was working opted out of the master agreement, laid off all the workers and hired them back at $15 an hour, with benefits cut sharply and workers forced to do split shifts. Many other care aides in the province were in the same boat, forced to work part-time and juggle shifts at several workplaces in order to make ends meet.

"Everything got cut. It didn't feel good, but you feel like you have no choice. You still have to feed your children," Marquez says. One study found that, on average, PSWs earn about $3,000 less a year than they did a decade ago. Casualization—the shift from full-time, permanent positions to casual and contract positions—has also become commonplace as employers look to cut benefits. Today, across Canada, only about 30 percent of care workers have full-time jobs, 40 percent work permanent part-time, and 30 percent are casuals. Many of the part-time and casual workers have jobs at more than one facility, or mix shifts at care homes with home care visits. It is not unusual for non-unionized care aides to work from 7 a.m. to 11 p.m., cramming in four-hour shifts at three different facilities, or six or more home visits. Care aides having to work at multiple facilities was one of the main reasons coronavirus spread like wildfire in care homes. When BC banned the practice, it was able to quell outbreaks quickly; Ontario and Quebec, because of the dire shortage of workers, allowed the practice to continue, and outbreaks lasted longer as a result.

When Marquez finally left the facility where she had worked for her entire career, in 2020, she was earning $21 an hour, including a night shift differential. (It is standard for unionized employees who work the night shift to get a premium, usually around 10 percent.) She returned to school part-time to study to be a licensed practical nurse, and took a job at a government-owned facility, which is still subject to the master agreement. As a care aide, she earns $25.45 an hour plus benefits, and that will increase slightly when she is licensed as an LPN.

Is that a fair wage?

"I don't think you can pay care aides enough for what they do," says Jennifer Whiteside, secretary–business manager of the BC Hospital Employees' Union. But she adds that she's not embarrassed to have negotiated the contract with the government, the most recent version of which was signed in March 2019. She notes that, in the private sector, there are workers getting as much as $7 an hour less for the same work. In some provinces, such as Quebec and Nova Scotia, workers are paid as little as $13 an hour, barely minimum wage. In many provinces there is also an entrenched hierarchy, where care aides in hospital get paid more than those in long-term-care facilities, who get more than those in nursing homes, with those in the home care sector paid the worst of all. "The work done by care aides is skilled and valuable regardless of where it's done, and they should be paid the same," Whiteside says.

While money is important, experts warn that hiking the pay of care aides will not, in itself, make care any better for patients, or necessarily improve the workplace. "Even if you give them an additional $10 an hour, if they don't have time to care for people properly, they won't necessarily do a better job," says Dr. Louis Demers, a professor at the École nationale d'administration publique in

Montreal. For that reason, Quebec has vowed to hire 10,000 new care workers in addition to the 40,000 it already has on the public payroll. All the new jobs will be in long-term-care homes. While that is an impressive political pledge, there are worries about the unintended consequences. Already, during the pandemic, PSWs jumped from the home care sector to the long-term-care sector because more hours were available and the pay was better, a classic case of robbing Peter to pay Paul. There are also concerns about attrition. It is one thing to offer free training and the promise of jobs; it is quite another for thousands of people who applied to stay committed once they recognize just how hard the work can be.

Dr. Demers says that people who simply want a pay cheque are not going to be good care workers, and given the rigours of the work, they're not going to last. People working in care homes (and home care) need to be sociable and conscientious and enjoy working with elders, he says. "It's not stocking shelves in a grocery store ... personal care workers are precious. They are important people and we have neglected them terribly."

While the bulk of hands-on care, about 90 percent, is done by PSWs, nurses also play a key role, and they too are in short supply and face similar challenges, including casualization and juggling part-time jobs. Over the years, as employers tried to keep their payrolls down, the number of registered nurses and LPNs has shrunk while their workload has grown tremendously. This has had an impact on patient care because nurses oversee the work of support staff, dispense medications—patients in care get a lot of prescription drugs—and are responsible for infection control. A typical long-term-care home will have only one RN per shift, and perhaps two LPNs, with all the other work done by care aides.

While a number of allied health professionals—rehabilitation therapists, occupational therapists, physical therapists, audiologists, speech-language pathologists and psychologists, to name a few—do a significant amount of work with elders, access to these specialized services varies greatly. Homes have a budget for support services, but it is allocated in different ways; provincial rules also vary on what ancillary services are covered. Homes also have a medical director, but that physician is rarely a full-time employee. Rather, despite the level of medical need, especially in long-term-care homes, the position is often viewed as a sinecure, awarded to retired physicians, some of whom are as old as the residents they treat. Some residents continue with their family doctor after admission, but few physicians do house calls; instead, they will call nurses with changes to medication and the like, a practice nurses derisively call "medicine by fax." Practically, when residents need even the most basic medical care, such as treatment of a urinary tract infection, they are shipped off to hospital emergency rooms. That's why, at almost every long-term-care facility, there is a steady flow of ambulances taking patients back and forth.

As the staffing issues have come under scrutiny, especially in long-term-care homes, there has been a growing push to legislate hours of care and staffing ratios to ensure that residents are getting adequate care. The Registered Nurses' Association of Ontario (RNAO) has led the charge in demanding a "basic care guarantee," calling for every resident of LTC to receive at least four hours daily of direct nursing and personal care. That number is based on work done by Charlene Harrington, professor emerita of sociology and nursing at the University of California, San Francisco, almost two decades ago. In a groundbreaking study that took five years of careful analysis of what care aides do, she found that it requires at least four hours to assist patients with basic activities of daily living. It's worth stressing that, since then, the population has aged markedly and patients have become more frail, their needs more complex.

Few care homes in Canada, whether they are government-owned, not-for-profit or for-profit, meet the four-hour standard now. The Ontario Long-Term Care Act states that every resident has the right to be properly sheltered, fed, clothed, groomed and cared for in a manner consistent with his or her needs; that every resident has the right to live in a safe and clean environment; and that every resident has the right to receive care and assistance based on a "restorative care" philosophy. The legislation is a behemoth of good intentions, backed up by a dizzying ninety-one pages of regulations, but nowhere does it set out either caregiver-to-patient ratios or a guarantee of minimum hours of care.

The BC Ministry of Health has had a standard of 3.36 hours of daily care per resident since 2008, but it is more aspiration than regulation. In a 2017 report, BC Seniors Advocate Isobel Mackenzie found that 91 percent of homes did not meet the standard. The problem, she wrote, is that "facilities are funded at levels that may not meet the guideline." In other words, it's not possible to provide the minimal standard of care with the money provided for staffing. "There's no way around it," Mackenzie said. "Fixing direct-care hours is going to cost money. It's about having the bodies there, and the bodies have to be paid."

According to the RNAO's analysis, Ontario fares even worse than BC, providing long-term-care residents with only 2.71 hours of hands-on care daily. That includes 0.3 hours of RN care, 0.49 hours from a registered practical nurse (RPN) and 1.92 hours from a PSW. That translates to a staffing mix of 11 percent RN, 18 percent RPN and 71 percent PSW. The RNAO, in its recommendation to government, said the proper mix should be 20 percent RN, 25 percent RPN and 55 percent PSW.

While there is broad support for guaranteeing a minimum level of care, many are reluctant to embrace the notion of precise minutes of care to be delivered by individual health workers because it risks degenerating into battles over turf protection and can be difficult to make work at the bedside. Then there's the money issue. Using the RNAO's formula would require the equivalent of more than 23,000 full-time workers in Ontario alone, including 9,000 RNs, 9,500 RPNs and 5,000 PSWs. That would cost the province an additional $1.8 billion a year.

Miranda Ferrier, national president of the Canadian Support Workers Association, says she prefers that ratios be established rather than hours/minutes of care to determine the number of staff needed. In research, there is a pretty broad consensus that 1:5 is a good ratio for care aides to patients in the average long-term-care home. In Canada, New Brunswick is the only province with that standard in its guidance. In practice, though, workers have much heavier workloads.

"We need to handle no more than six to eight patients [per shift] to make the job bearable for workers and the care decent for residents," Ferrier says. "Right now, PSWs are handling twelve to twenty patients, and that's not good for anyone."

Addressing wage disparities, staff mix and ratios will be an enormous task for governments, employers, unions and associations, but there is also a need to tackle how care aides are educated and regulated.

Unlike medicine, nursing and allied professions, there is no national educational standard for PSWs. There are excellent 32-week college programs. But courses are offered in a wide variety of settings, including community colleges, career colleges and vocational programs offered at high schools, and they vary in quality, length and cost. There are also online programs that are little more than diploma mills. "I had someone send me their credentials and they had literally 'graduated' from Bob's School of PSWs," Ferrier says. When Quebec made its much-publicized pledge to hire ten thousand care workers in June 2020, it promised a "fast-tracked" twelve-week training program, during which students would be paid $760 a week, followed by a guaranteed full-time position in a CHSLD at $49,000 a year when they graduated. Time will tell whether this sped-up cohort of orderlies will be up to the task when they get out into the real world, and whether they are in it for the long haul.

Because it is not a regulated profession, anyone can call themselves a care aide or PSW or whatever designation they choose. That can make it difficult for employers who are desperate for workers, as well as for families, who are increasingly hiring help under the table. Ferrier says the lack of regulation is a fundamental flaw that needs to be fixed for the sake of workers, employers and patients. "If I put all the issues in our profession up on a white-board—and there are a lot of them—the one that would be on top is self-regulation," Ferrier says. "If we want to fix everything else, we need self-regulation that comes with it."

Provincial governments let certain professions self-regulate, meaning they can establish entry requirements, professional standards and appropriate discipline. The central purpose is to ensure public safety, the idea being that, for example, physicians will not tolerate an incompetent colleague because it will besmirch the entire profession. Oversight is provided by a college, ideally with public representatives on the board and present in disciplinary hearings.

In Ontario, there are twenty-seven regulated health professions, from audiology, chiropody and dental hygiene to speech-language pathology, traditional Chinese medicine and acupuncture. There are just three non-regulated health professions: PSWs, physician assistants and physiotherapy assistants. "It's absurd," Ferrier says, noting that people who clean your teeth have stricter standards oversight than those who care for some of the most vulnerable people in society—elders living in care homes.

Because government has resisted creating a College of Personal Support Workers, the Canadian Support Workers Association created its own informal body called the Personal Support Workers Institute of Canada. In Ontario, Saskatchewan and Newfoundland and Labrador—the three provinces that use the designation PSW—the institute will verify the credentials of PSWs, do a criminal record check and ensure they have $1 million in liability insurance. The informal system also allows members of the public to check that workers are legit and file complaints that will be investigated. However, joining the PSW association and respecting the college's rulings are purely voluntary.

Not everyone thinks self-regulation is a priority, or especially important. "Creating a college and more formal regulation is not going to make life any better for residents," Jennifer Whiteside of the BC Hospital Employees' Union insists. "We need nurses to do what they're trained to do and we need care aides to do what they're trained to do."

BC has a standard education curriculum and a care aide registry, and there's no reason other provinces can't do the same, she says. (Ontario has twice tried to create a registry and both times it flopped, largely because the issue became highly politicized.) Whiteside believes the priority should be unionization of workers, which would create a better work environment and, by extension, improved care for patients in LTC and home care. She notes that eldercare was horrible until the 1970s, when workers began organizing and the government started imposing standards. When there was a flurry of contracting out and union busting in the early

2000s, care once again deteriorated, creating a "perfect storm" of conditions for the coronavirus to ravage the residents of care homes. "Unionization formalizes the structure and relationship between employers and workers. It creates a safe venue for raising issues about the quality of care and the work environment," Whiteside says.

Beyond the technical debates about self-regulation versus unionization, and the political discussions about funding and staffing, there is a much more important societal debate to be had about values, and what we value, according to Whiteside. The structure and culture of eldercare sends the implicit message that once you reach a certain age, or a certain degree of disability, you cease to be useful or valued, and that seems un-Canadian, she adds. "Do we want to just maintain seniors until they die, or do we want to create environments where they can have the best quality of life possible for the time they have left?

"This is why staffing matters. This is why ratios matter. If we really value seniors, if we really respect our elders, then we have to start with that values proposition."

CHAPTER 7

Conscripted by Love

The struggle to balance caring for children and caring for aging parents is what defines the sandwich generation. It's a group made up almost exclusively of middle-aged working women, over-extended and being squeezed increasingly tighter as child-bearing is delayed and their own parents (and in-laws) live longer and require more care. Sylvie Guibert could have been the sandwich generation's meme, always seeking that ever-elusive work–life balance under the weight of her caregiving duties. At age 49, she was working full-time, mother to two active teenagers and caring for her ailing 89-year-old mother-in-law, who had moved into the family home.

Then, one morning, as they were still lying in bed, her husband, Jacques Farley, suffered a massive hemorrhagic stroke, where a weak blood vessel bursts and bleeds into the brain. Only about one in four people survive this type of catastrophic bleed. While Jacques did survive, he was left with significant disability, paralyzed down the left side of his body, with his foot remaining upturned, which made walking very difficult. The damage to his brain also robbed him of most short-term memory and changed his personality significantly.

The happy, comfortable family suddenly saw their lives turned upside down. Jacques spent eight months in rehabilitation at Ottawa's St. Vincent Hospital, where Sylvie visited him daily. Her mother-in-law's health declined precipitously and she died two months into the ordeal.

While stroke rehab can sometimes work miracles, it was becoming clear that Jacques's paralysis was likely permanent; he would probably never walk unassisted again, and the pain he suffered would be chronic. At age 55, he was never going to return to work either. His progress in rehab had plateaued, so it was time for Jacques to be discharged. A life-altering decision needed to be made: would he return home or be transferred to a long-term-care facility?

The decision to care for someone who needs assistance 24/7 is not one to be taken lightly, especially for someone with numerous work and family obligations, but Sylvie was offered little guidance. "I went the bring-him-home route and no one discouraged me, or explained to me just how much work it would be," she says. It seemed the hospital's priority was freeing up a bed, not providing information or counselling. "I thought bringing him home would provide some stability and maybe help with his rehab. I guess I was a bit naive." Knowing what she knows now, she admits she's not sure she would have made the same choice.

"Don't get me wrong, I love my husband and I'm happy we had all those years together as a family. But I'm not going to lie, it was hard, it was really, really hard." It was long too. Sylvie would spend eleven and a half years as her husband's principal, and often sole, caregiver.

At some point, almost every Canadian will become a caregiver. The demands may be short-term and straightforward or, as for

Sylvie Guibert, intense and long-term. Caregiving duties span a vast gamut of physical, emotional and financial assistance, or any combination thereof. And, as the population ages and the pool of caregivers shrinks, we will all almost certainly be called upon to help a loved one at least once—or twice, or multiple times.

Currently, about one in four Canadians over the age of 15—or 7.8 million people—provide care to a family member or friend with a "long-term health condition, a physical or mental disability, or problems related to aging," according to Statistics Canada. Almost half of all caregivers, 47 percent, care primarily for parents or parents-in-law. (The majority are in the 45-to-54 demographic, the sandwich generation.) Another 13 percent care for a spouse or partner, and most of this group are seniors themselves. The 55-year-old daughter caring for her 85-year-old mother is commonplace; so too is an 88-year-old wife acting as the primary caregiver for her 88-year-old husband. But not everyone has family to step up, or a spouse. Thirteen percent of caregivers take care of a friend or neighbour, 10 percent a sibling, 9 percent a grandparent. Another 8 percent are primary caregivers for a child with a serious physical, developmental or psychiatric disability, and they often perform these duties for decades.

The Statistics Canada data tell us that 54 percent of caregivers are women and 46 percent are men. But the appearance of "close to gender parity" is misleading, because the care women provide is far more intense and intimate. It may seem stereotypical, but the reality is that men generally cover tasks such as paying the bills and cutting the lawn, while women do hands-on care such as bathing and toileting. Women also carry out a lot of duties that don't really show up in the statistics, such as checking in and planning. They also tend to do the tasks that can't wait, so there's far less flexibility as to when they are done. Not to mention that women still do a disproportionate amount of domestic chores and caring for children. Women are even less likely to identify themselves as caregivers, because caring for parents or spouses is often seen as a normal part of the continuum of unpaid care throughout women's lives. As Sylvie Guibert puts it, "You do what you have to do." Like Sylvie, most take on caregiving duties willingly, but also feel conscripted to care by the lack of viable alternatives, and unsupported by the health and social welfare systems when they need help.

Caregivers can have vastly different levels of engagement. Almost half of the 7.8 million carers provide only a few hours of care a week, which can involve running errands or helping with housework. But one in four caregivers contribute more than twenty hours of care weekly, and one in ten have duties that take forty hours a week or more—in other words, more than a full-time job. And as if that were not enough, caregiving usually begins suddenly, with no prior notice.

"Despite little to no training, [caregivers] are expected to provide medical and nursing care in the home, navigate complicated health and long-term-care systems, and serve as substitute decision-makers," says Dr. Nathan Stall, a geriatrician and research fellow at Women's College Research Institute. Caregivers need training, he explains, because they do a lot more than cooking and dusting; bathing someone frail requires skill, as does changing the incontinence pad of an unco-operative adult. One in five family members provide advanced medical care, including changing gastrostomy tubes, dressing wounds and giving injections.

"Most Canadian caregivers do not have access to caregiver-specific education and supports despite evidence that these can improve their well-being and that of the care recipient," Dr. Stall points out.

A good example of caregiver training and support is a program called CARERS (coaching, advocacy, respite, education, relationship, simulation) offered by the Cyril & Dorothy, Joel & Jill Reitman Centre at Mount Sinai Hospital in Toronto. The ten-session program, offered free of charge to caregivers of elders with dementia being treated at the hospital, is designed to equip family members with practical skills and emotional supports, using professional actors to simulate all manner of challenging situations. The course—a variation of which is also offered in the workplace by some large employers—has been shown to give caregivers more confidence and significantly reduce both burnout and the rate of injury in dementia patients. (The care recipients meet separately with an occupational therapist and also learn coping skills.)

Dr. Stall says the CARERS program is the "gold standard" and demonstrates the benefits and necessity of training. "While caregiving for older adults can be rewarding, it is increasingly demanding, complex and stressful," he explains, and caregivers need all the support they can get. Offering to teach people practical skills also results in the burden of care being shared more equally among family members, even though it is usually assumed that women are imbued with these "soft skills." One-third of women with parents over the age of 65 take time off work to fulfill caregiving duties; others sacrifice sleep, a social life, and physical and mental health to keep working and carry out caregiving duties at the same time.

In Sylvie Guibert's case, she was determined to keep working full-time, for a couple of reasons. As a federal government employee, she had an excellent benefits package, including a prescription drug plan and physiotherapy coverage, which helped with her husband's medical needs. She also needed the income to support her family, and wanted to ensure she would receive a full pension so she could continue to do so in the future.

The most common form of financial aid for caregivers is tax relief, but it is usually distributed as refundable tax credits, and they are only beneficial if you have a substantial income. As a result, only a tiny minority receive tax credits. Low-income caregivers have almost no support; the exception is in Nova Scotia, where they are eligible for a monthly benefit similar to social assistance. This lack of financial support means that people end up in LTC earlier, even if they have family members who are willing to provide care at home.

There is also a compassionate care benefit, where caregivers can get up to six months of Employment Insurance benefits to care for a critically ill or dying family member. But such programs tend to be very narrowly focused and difficult to navigate. For example, the compassionate care benefit is only available if the person being cared for is at imminent risk of death. Most people with chronic illness have recurrent exacerbations over long periods. What most caregivers need are direct reimbursements or allowances for out-of-pocket costs.

In Sylvie's case, her husband, Jacques, had significant disabilities, but his condition was stable and he was relatively young, so there was little home care help available from the publicly funded health system—just a few hours a week. Managing that was often more trouble than it was worth, because workers routinely showed up late, if at all, and that would throw a wrench into the workday. Sylvie ended up hiring a PSW, Jovencio Omapas. That young man became a mainstay of care for more than five years, tending to Jacques's needs from 8 a.m. to 5 p.m. daily so that Sylvie could get her work done.

But hiring a full-time employee—Jovencio was a Filipino man who came to Canada as part of the Temporary Foreign Worker Program—also entailed significant bureaucratic work and, because he lived in an apartment in the basement, there was another mouth to feed. As Sylvie describes the situation, "I had to apply for a permit, learn to do payroll and other things. The worst part was Revenue Canada treated me like a business. It's not like I was making a profit caring for my husband—on the contrary!"

While we talk a lot about the role of physicians, nurses, PSWs and allied health professionals, the reality is that the vast majority of eldercare is done by unpaid caregivers. If their unpaid labour were remunerated at the equivalent of minimum wage (say $14 an hour), it would be worth somewhere between $26 billion and $72 billion a year, according to a study by the Change Foundation. Caregivers also rack up about $6 billion a year in out-of-pocket costs, and that includes only direct spending, not foregone wages, benefits and pension entitlement.

Sylvie never calculated exactly how much she spent over more than a decade of care, but it was significant, more than $30,000 a year when she had a live-in care aide, and at least $10,000 a year when she was alone at home, and that only includes the amounts she was able to claim for tax purposes. "How did I pay for all this? I worked, and I indebted the family," she says. "I used the equity in the house to pay for my husband's care until my retirement, then I sold the house to pay our debts."

Caregiving is not only financially, physically and mentally taxing, it has an impact on the family dynamic. Sylvie was determined to keep the family together, but she recognizes now that the situation was especially hard on their children, Julie-Anne and Marie-Lyne. "In many ways, they lost their father. Everything was focused on his needs," she observes. Making matters worse, the neurological damage Jacques suffered meant his long-term memories were intact but not his short-term memory. "In his mind he remembered them as babies, and he never adjusted to them growing up, and that was always difficult for the kids." The brain damage from the stroke also meant that a once-kind man no longer had any empathy, so he provided no emotional support to his children and often appeared uncaring.

Sylvie was the principal breadwinner in the family. Her husband received disability insurance payments, but those ended when he turned 65 and became eligible for old age security, which meant $800 less a month in income. When Sylvie took an early retirement, at age 55 (after thirty-seven years in the public service), her income dropped, so she had to lay off Jovencio. She became her husband's sole caregiver, and it was a demanding 24/7 job.

Jacques lived with chronic pain, and that entailed a lot of medical appointments. A big man at five foot nine and over two hundred pounds, he needed to be helped, physically, to get out of bed or to the bathroom, and he didn't like using a wheelchair because it exacerbated his pain. "It's really physically demanding care," Sylvie says. It was also relentless. "Once the kids moved out to go to school, I was alone and I could barely leave the house for an hour. I would be doing groceries and he would call and say, 'I have to go to the bathroom.'"

Sylvie continues, "Being on the clock like that for five years— you can't imagine how tiring and stressful that is." She says it was years before she discovered, quite by accident, that there is something called respite care—temporary institutional care to provide a break for people caring for loved ones at home. "They really don't tell you anything," she says.

But Sylvie learned that respite care can sound a lot better than it is. Preparing her husband to be away from her for a couple of weeks took a lot of effort, and then her holiday was hardly relaxing. "It would take me at least a week to unwind, and mostly I would sleep, then I would spend the next week stressing about all the things I would have to do when I got back."

Jacques had his stroke in April 2008. In May 2019, Sylvie decided she was no longer able to care for him at home. More precisely, her doctor convinced her. "She kept saying to me: 'Sylvie, you're exhausted. You're going to end up in the hospital. Then what?'"

While the wait list for placement in LTC is long, Jacques was lucky, waiting only six months for a spot and ending up with his first choice, Élisabeth Bruyère Residence, where they found the care to be first-rate. Sylvie still visits her husband almost every day—or at least she did until pandemic restrictions shut out care-givers and visitors alike. Jacques was infected with coronavirus but didn't get too ill and recovered fairly quickly. But the lockdown, which lasted more than five months, was devastating to residents, leaving many dangerously inactive and isolated. During this period, Jacques became increasingly bed-bound. Because he is much bigger and heavier than most residents, staff use a lift to get him out of bed and he feels he is being a bother, so he eats in bed rather than the dining room, and participates in few activities. When the lock-down lifted, however, Sylvie insisted he get out and about more, and that he go outside for the first time in almost half a year—just another example that underscores how important the presence of caregivers is, even in "full-service" facilities.

On her daily visits, Sylvie cleans up her husband's room, assists him with eating and dressing, helps him to the bathroom and pro-vides companionship. While she has nothing but praise for the nurses and PSWs, the reality is that, with the staffing levels that exist, they can't possibly give every resident the attention they deserve.

"If Jacques drops his fork, he'll have to wait an hour for some-one to pick it up. That seems like a petty thing, but when there aren't enough workers, the residents lose out on quality of life," Sylvie says.

Jacques, at 67, is, by LTC standards, a young man. While he has physical disabilities, he has no cognitive issues. Because he's aware of what's going on, Sylvie says life in institutional care is a lot more difficult. "He will ring the bell to go to the bathroom and they'll say: 'We don't have time. Just go in your diaper and we'll clean you up later.' Imagine if you had to live your life like that. It's not dignified."

Dignity and quality of life are the exact reasons Deiren Masterson chose to care for his parents at home. When his mom, Maureen, was diagnosed with Parkinson's disease at age 84, he returned from where he was living in the UK to help with her care. His father, Paul, 86, was already suffering from chronic obstructive pulmonary disease and heart problems (he had both a cardiac pacemaker and an implantable cardioverter-defibrillator) and couldn't take care of his wife alone. Deiren arrived just in time: his mom began falling often and she was in and out of hospital. When Maureen broke her shoulder in a particularly bad fall, she was admitted to hospital, which turned into a nightmarish two-week ordeal. She developed delirium, a state of confused thinking that often occurs with elders who are hospitalized, especially after surgery. "She went downhill really fast. She stopped eating. She was agitated, so they prescribed her an antipsychotic to calm her and instead it threw her into chaos," Deiren recalls. "Suddenly she didn't know I was her son. She was screaming: 'Who are you? Who are you?'"

That cascade of physical and mental health problems related to delirium is shockingly common. Delirium rates range from 11 to 65 percent on hospital wards. It is largely avoidable if patients sleep well, eat well, and are physically and mentally active, all things that rarely happen in busy hospitals, especially when there's no advocate or caregiver nearby. Deiren decided to stay with his mother around the clock, even sleeping on the floor of her hospital room.

The treating physician recommended that Maureen be transferred immediately to a long-term-care home, a crisis placement. Her husband had no idea what to do; like many couples, they had never discussed these all-important matters. Even though they were in their 80s and had a plethora of serious health issues between them, the Mastersons had not prepared advance directives, do-not-resuscitate orders or power of attorney. They had never talked about what would happen if one or both of them developed serious mental or physical disability and needed institutional care. Those are difficult but essential conversations, best done when people are healthy and lucid, not in times of crisis.

Deiren took charge. "I said, 'No way, we're taking her home.' They really pushed for long-term care, but I knew that's not what she wanted." The family scrambled to rent a hospital bed and arrange for a nurse to visit to do wound care on the serious pressure ulcer (bedsore) Maureen had developed in hospital. For the next two years, the bulk of the care was done by Deiren, with help from one of his sisters. Throughout the ordeal, he worked, but decided to only take contracts so he would have as much time as possible as a caregiver. To add to the stress, his wife, who is Italian, was still overseas much of that time, but finally managed to get approval to immigrate.

Unlike many sons, Deiren was not only willing but able to provide care to his mom. When he was younger, he had worked as a live-in assistant in the community of L'Arche Daybreak in Richmond Hill, Ontario, where he provided support for residents with severe physical and developmental disabilities.

"At L'Arche, the training and experience was incredible. We did everything except emergency medical care, so I wasn't really afraid of anything when it came to dealing with my parents," Deiren explains. "I was also trained to be an advocate, and that's probably the number one skill you need as a caregiver."

After his mother came home from hospital, his father's health also declined steadily, and he was in and out of hospital. Caregiving became more than a full-time job, and there was never more than fifteen hours weekly of home care offered to the two parents combined. Deiren and the family came to the painful realization that the "home where my parents had spent their entire married life and raised their eight children was no longer suitable." It's a decision that many families have to make and, again, it's best to prepare a transition plan when everyone is of sound mind and body, not when there are many other daily challenges to manage.

The Mastersons decided to move into a retirement home and hire PSWs to come in and supplement the care provided by their children. But that arrangement lasted only a few months. A severe flu outbreak hit the nursing home—a reminder that infectious disease challenges existed before coronavirus. Both Paul and Maureen ended up in hospital, the latter gravely ill in the intensive care unit. Once Maureen's life was out of danger, she was transferred to a long-term-care facility, an emergency placement she had avoided nearly two years earlier. This time the family didn't resist. Paul Masterson decided to follow his wife so they could be together.

"The long-term-care home my parents ended up in was actually nice. It was a private room, it had big windows, and a faith element that was important to them," Deiren says. "But you soon realize that, even in the best places, you don't get the attention and the care you should. You have to supplement their care. There's no way around it. I could accept my parents dying of illness, but I could not accept them dying of neglect."

The children hired PSWs to care for their parents during the day. They did this, ironically, to provide stability; there was constant turnover in the staff at the home, but the caregivers hired privately stayed on long-term. Deiren also wanted to ensure there was a strong, respectful relationship between care provider and patient, something he learned was essential during his time at L'Arche. "The PSWs didn't do just tasks, they provided companionship, emotional and spiritual support. They became part of the family."

Deiren was working full-time at this point, but each day after work he went directly to the home, and stayed from 4:30 p.m. until 9 p.m., helping with dinner and preparations for bedtime. His father died after only a few months in the home; he never fully recovered from a severe case of influenza, which greatly exacerbated his COPD. But his mother lived another year before she too died.

"You ended up doing things you never expected. Changing your mom's diapers is hard. But the alternative is having her sit in wet Depends for hours waiting for someone else to do it." While family members who take a hands-on role in care lessen the burden on PSWs in care homes, Deiren says they didn't really appreciate him and his sister being around. He felt they were treated as a bother rather than an essential part of the care equation.

The demands on caregivers go down when loved ones are in LTC, but the financial requirements increase. "We're certainly not the Kennedys, but we found the money," Deiren says. "It was important for us to care for our parents as best we could. That's more important than an inheritance."

While their experiences were markedly different, Deiren Masterson and Sylvie Guibert have similar advice for people with elderly parents who are slowly creeping up in age, and it can be summarized in two words: *be prepared.*

Nobody likes to talk about the fact that they could end up with a severe disability or a partner who needs round-the-clock care, but having those uncomfortable conversations can really take a lot of pressure off caregivers later on. No caregiver will ever complain about getting crystal-clear direction—in the form of advance directives, power of attorney and stated preferences. Should the family home be sold if Mom develops dementia and needs to go into LTC? That kind of discussion should happen when the homeowner is compos mentis, not when they've started wandering dangerously.

Both caregivers also stressed the need to be fully informed of options before making key decisions, such as choosing between home care and institutional care, or whether to take a leave from work. The health and social welfare systems do a terrible job of conveying basic information and often rush families to decide. "You have to push back. You have to be an advocate for your loved ones," Deiren Masterson says.

You also have to advocate for and care for yourself. Older caregivers often fall ill after the death of their partner. Younger caregivers burn out. There are warnings signs to watch for: overwhelming fatigue, sleep problems, feeling as though caregiving is controlling your life, depression, and difficulty coping with everyday tasks. Experts urge caregivers to reach out to friends, family, peer support groups. They also caution that, at a certain point, you may have to say, "*No mas*." Of course, that isn't easy. But, as Sylvie Guibert's doctor told her, if you work yourself to death, your loved one will be worse off.

Finally, there needs to be a broad societal discussion about the realities of caregiving, about the expectations that are and will continue to be placed on the shrinking pool of caregivers as the number of those needing care increases. We have to start caring for our caregivers. But we also need to prepare them for what is expected of them. In Sylvie Guibert's words, "No one grows up thinking: 'I'm going to be a caregiver someday, for my husband, my in-laws, my parents.' But maybe we should think about those things a little more."

CHAPTER 8

This Is the End

All that lives must die, passing through nature to eternity.

—WILLIAM SHAKESPEARE,
Hamlet, Act 1, Scene 2

Every year, about one in every hundred Canadians dies. More than 80 percent of those deaths are among people over the age of 65.

For elders, death is very much part of life. There is a reason they are avid readers of the obituaries. Yet, in our death-denying society, we do little to prepare our elders for death, and even less to ensure they have a dignified death.

Fewer than one in three Canadians have access to palliative care at the end of life. There are pockets of excellence, like palliative care for patients with cancer and AIDS. But there are also areas where we fail miserably at palliation, notably for patients with dementia and others living in long-term-care facilities, who too often suffer unduly. While home care is inadequate for the living, it is doubly so for the dying. Only one in six Canadians can get palliative care at home. Fewer still can find a place in hospice at the end of life. Access depends largely on happenstance.

"Everyone should have a choice of where they die," says Dr. Darren Cargill, medical director of the Hospice of Windsor and Essex County. "Unfortunately, they don't. It's a postal code lottery."

Since our health system is hospital-centric, most deaths happen there by default, Dr. Cargill notes—this despite the fact that surveys show, time and time again, that hospital is the last place people want to spend their final days and hours. They prefer home, or a homelike environment such as hospice.

Bill Major made his choice clear years ago, when he was diagnosed with COPD. When his health deteriorated greatly in December 2018, he reiterated that choice: home was where he was going to live out his final days, and home was where he was going to die.

"Long-term care was never an option for Poppa, and Nana wouldn't hear of it either. Come hell or high water, he was going to stay at home," recalls Melissa Bonafazi, his granddaughter.

Bill did stay at home until July 2020, with the help of family caregivers and a bit of home care. As a veteran of the Korean War, he was entitled to more home care and support services than most, and that helped. But during the pandemic, home care services were cut drastically out of fear that PSWs could spread coronavirus to patients, so even more of the burden fell on his wife, Marilyn, 84. As care demands grew, the doting spouse suffered both physically and psychologically.

One night, as Bill was experiencing increasingly frequent bouts of delirium, Marilyn cracked and called 911. When the paramedics arrived, they were going to transport him to hospital but noticed that he had both do-not-resuscitate and do-not-hospitalize orders by his bed. So they called other family members, who in turn contacted the local hospice.

"ER is the absolute worse place to die," insists Melissa. "We had talked about that, but my grandmother sort of panicked [when she called 911] because she was overwhelmed, something she had kept a secret."

Instead of sending Bill to the ER, where no useful medical care could be provided and where patients' delirium often grows far worse, the family rallied to keep him at home. A home care nurse provided palliative care on an emergency basis, and then, when a bed became available, Bill was transferred to hospice. There, he spent the final three days of his life, and died on July 24 at age 87.

Bill Major had a good death: his symptoms were controlled, his pain was minimized, he had constant, specialized nursing care, and he was surrounded by family. He also had every advantage. Unlike most people, Bill and Marilyn had planned meticulously for their eventual demise. They made their end-of-life wishes clear to family, and prepared legal documents such as advanced directives, DNRs and DNHs. The couple even chose their plots and head-stones, paid for in advance. They also had an ace up their sleeve: Melissa was not only a loving granddaughter but also a palliative care nurse at the Hospice of Windsor.

"I've done this many times as a nurse, but as a family member the experience was surreal," she says. "A lot of people are lost when they try to get help for their loved ones. The system really doesn't make it easy. If I didn't have the background and knowledge that I do, I have no doubt Poppa's death would have been a nightmare."

As a frustrated family member, Melissa observed, as many expert reports have noted over the years, that the system's short-comings, from lack of navigation to inadequate home care ser-vices, push every patient to the most impersonal and expensive options: LTC and hospital.

Dr. Cargill says the fundamental problem with palliative care in Canada—aside from the obvious lack of resources—is cultural, a lack of willingness to discuss and plan for death, both on an individual and on a societal level. "Way too many people are falling through cracks at the end of life. When someone dies poorly, it reinforces the fear of death and dying. It's a vicious circle," he says.

About 285,000 people die in Canada each year, and that number will increase to more than 430,000 within two decades. In an aging society, improving the end-of-life experience should be a priority for a host of reasons—financial, medical and ethical.

But what is a good death? Researchers at the University of California, San Diego School of Medicine compiled findings from mountains of research carried out with patients, family members and care providers and identified several key conditions associated with dying well. The three most important, mentioned by virtually everyone, were: 1) being in control, specifically having their wishes on where and how they die respected; 2) being pain-free; and 3) having quality of life, or enjoying the time they have left to the fullest. Other issues identified included feeling a sense that life is complete, having their religious beliefs respected, having a good relationship with care providers, and being able to make choices about treatments. Finally, being with family and able to say goodbye to loved ones mattered a lot.

Dr. Cargill, who has been a palliative care physician for more than fifteen years, says every one of those factors can come into play to varying degrees but there is no single way of ensuring a perfect end. "A good death means different things to different people. But the one thing everyone wants is a dignified death. For that to happen, people have to plan and we have to respect their choices."

In Canadian health care, choices are rarely offered, and that is particularly true at the end of life. There is a dire shortage of specialists in palliative care, so it is provided by family physicians, who have very little training in pain management. (One study found Canadian veterinary students received five times more training in pain management than Canadian medical students.) When patients are in hospital, they are cared for by nurses and doctors whose priority is keeping them alive, not ensuring a peaceful passing. When patients' wishes are not explicit, they can undergo a lot of procedures that prolong their life but also prolong their suffering. Hospital rooms tend to be loud, bright and hectic, the very opposite of peaceful. Transfers to the hospital's palliative unit—if there even is one—often don't happen until the last minute, if at all.

To make matters worse, there is no consensus on what receiving palliative care means and what services this should include. That makes it a challenge to determine when palliative care should begin, how to set standards of care and what data should be collected.

However, the World Health Organization has identified the elements of good palliative care:

- provides relief from pain and other distressing symptoms;
- affirms life and regards dying as a normal process;
- intends neither to hasten nor postpone death;
- integrates the psychological and spiritual aspects of patient care;
- offers a support system to help patients live as actively as possible until death;
- offers a support system to help the family cope during the patient's illness and in their own bereavement;
- uses a team approach to address the needs of patients and their families, including bereavement counselling, if indicated;
- will enhance quality of life and may also positively influence the course of illness; and
- is applicable early in the course of illness, in conjunction with other therapies that are intended to prolong life, such as

chemotherapy or radiation therapy, and includes those investigations needed to better understand and manage distressing
clinical complications.

Dr. Cargill observes that regardless of the definition we use for palliative care, it is important to address a number of myths and mis-
understandings that exist. "Palliative care is not about giving up, it's
about improving your quality of life for the time you have left. The
other big myth is that we stop treating patients. We don't. We use
treatments that are appropriate. A lot of my cancer patients are on
chemo even if they are dying. And, of course, we do pain control."

Studies show that between 62 and 89 percent of people could
benefit from palliative care at the end of life—virtually everyone
who doesn't die unexpectedly. And, despite what we see on TV
every day—people being shot, getting blown up, crashing in planes
and so on—the vast majority of deaths are neither sudden nor violent. Rather, most people die from chronic illnesses such as cancer
and cardiovascular disease, and the course of illness is often quite
predictable.

THE 10 LEADING CAUSES OF DEATH IN CANADA

CAUSE	ANNUAL DEATHS	% OF ALL DEATHS
Cancer	79,536	28.0%
Cardiovascular diseases	53,134	18.7%
Stroke	13,480	4.8%
Unintentional injuries	13,290	4.7%
Respiratory diseases	12,998	4.6%
Influenza/pneumonia	8,511	3.0%
Diabetes	6,794	2.4%

CAUSE	ANNUAL DEATHS	% OF ALL DEATHS
Dementia	6,429	2.3%
Suicide	3,811	1.3%
Kidney disease	3,615	1.3%

Virtually everyone living in long-term-care facilities suffers from at least one of these chronic conditions, and often several. Yet access to palliative care is even worse in institutional settings than in the community. Only 6 percent of long-term-care residents get palliative care, according to data published by the Canadian Institute for Health Information. And that figure predates the coronavirus pandemic, when thousands of patients died without even basic end-of-life care. In its damning reports of conditions in long-term-care facilities hit hard by Covid-19, the Canadian Forces singled out "poor palliative care" as a major failing, saying dying residents did not benefit even from simple gestures such as moistening dry mouths and wiping away tears.

The lack of proper palliative measures in institutional care is not only shocking but counterintuitive. Long-term care is their last home for virtually everyone who is admitted. There is scarcely a resident who has a condition that is curable or even effectively treatable. In fact, on average, residents die within eighteen months of admission to LTC. But most residents who are in the final stages of death are transferred to hospital because institutional staff are not trained in palliative care and their patient loads are too heavy to permit them to provide that care.

Logically, we should be operating long-term-care facilities with a palliative care approach, as glorified hospices if you will, says Dr. Janice Legere, medical director of John Noble Home in Brantford, Ontario. "This is not the time for heroic measures and unnecessary trips to hospitals that often fail to extend life and instead cause more suffering and complications. It is a time to focus on living as well as possible until the end of life, based on an individual's values and needs."

Dr. Legere, a family physician with a passion for palliative care, says the priority for every resident of LTC should be advance care planning, a process of thinking about and writing down your wishes or instructions for present or future health care treatment, and drafting clear goals of care. "The most important thing is to talk to residents and family about what kind of care they want— something really aggressive, [or] comfort care, or some hybrid, illness by illness."

She stresses that comfort care, or palliative care, is *not* "not treating," but rather ensuring there is no unnecessary treatment. "It is not a resignation or a giving-in to death; instead, it is embracing life and all that we are—physically, emotionally, socially, psychologically and spiritually," Dr. Legere explains.

People who get palliative care not only live better, they live longer. They also require a lot less medical care at the end of life— fewer emergency room visits, fewer hospital admissions, less surgery, and less time spent in intensive care and critical care units.

Dame Cicely Saunders, a British nurse, is credited with the creation of the modern hospice movement. In 1948, she fell in love with a patient who was dying of cancer, and after his death she dedicated herself to learning about pain control and the grieving process. She spent many years ruminating on the idea before opening the now-legendary St. Christopher's Hospice in London in 1967, where the philosophy of care was: "You matter because you are you, you matter to the last moment of your life." Along the way, Dame Cicely studied to become a physician and grew profoundly religious. She had many devoted followers, one of whom was Dr. Balfour Mount, a urologist and professor at McGill University in Montreal.

He is credited with coining the term "palliative care" during a study he conducted of terminally ill patients at Montreal's Royal Victoria Hospital. In 1975, Dr. Mount launched Canada's first palliative care program at the Royal Vic.

Britain has kept Dame Cicely's legacy alive. It is widely considered the best place in the world to die. In fact, the Quality of Death Index, which ranks countries according to their provision of end-of-life care, ranks the UK as number one. It takes hospice and palliative care seriously. The National Health Service has decided, as a matter of public policy, that the quality of death is as important as the quality of life. The care itself is good and publicly funded. Health care providers are trained in palliation, painkillers are used liberally at the end of life, and there is a high degree of doctor–patient transparency (meaning the wishes of patients and families are respected).

Canada, despite Dr. Mount's pioneering efforts, didn't fare so well on the index, ranking ninth. Canada is renowned for its technical abilities—using medication and other techniques such as music therapy to lessen pain and suffering—but scored poorly because of chronic access problems. End-of-life care in this country is poorly coordinated, so access is uneven. (If you're wondering, the best places to die in Canada are Victoria, Edmonton and Windsor.) Palliative care is also expensive in Canada, largely because many services and drugs needed at the end of life are not covered by medicare. Patient-centred care is lacking, meaning patients' wishes are not respected nearly enough. Finally, there is an absence of policy leadership, with a few exceptions, such as the tireless work of Sharon Carstairs, who served briefly as the minister responsible for palliative care in Prime Minister Jean Chrétien's cabinet and advocated for better end-of-life care for many years as a senator.

The Canadian Hospice Palliative Care Association, in a 2010 report entitled *Quality of End-of-Life Care? It Depends on Where You Live . . . and Where You Die*, said end-of-life care in Canada "needs to be fixed from the ground up." The CHPCA said there are four essential components to making end-of-life care an integral part of medicare:

- *Universality*: Everyone nearing the end of life needs psychological, spiritual and physical support that is affordable.
- *Coordinated care*: In Canada, different aspects of care tend to operate in silos, and end-of-life care becomes an afterthought.
- *A broad range of services*: The needs of the dying vary widely, and hospice/palliative care should come in many forms.
- *Provision of care regardless of setting*: End-of-life care should be available in the family home, nursing homes, acute-care hospitals and hospices, and patients should have choice.

The issue of choice has come to the forefront of end-of-life discussions in recent years as Canada became one of only six countries in the world to legalize physician-assisted death (referred to in Canada by the acronym MAID, for "medical assistance in dying"). The change was a long time coming. Sue Rodriguez, a BC woman who suffered from ALS (Lou Gehrig's disease), challenged the ban on assisted suicide (as it was then referred to in the law) in 1991, asking famously: "If I cannot give consent to my own death, whose body is this? Who owns my life?" The Supreme Court rejected her constitutional challenge, but the court revisited the issue in 2015 and struck down the prohibition.

Most chronically ill patients die in a process known formally as "voluntary stopping of eating and drinking," or VSED. As a disease progresses, for example if their heart is failing, a person loses their desire to eat and drink, and their organs shut down. A variation on this is "withdrawing of potentially life-saving treatment," something crudely referred to as "pulling the plug." In these cases, a patient may require mechanical ventilation, or extracorporeal membrane oxygenation (ECMO), a fancy term for a heart-and-lung machine, and if there is no prospect of recovery the treatment can be discontinued. Both these approaches result in a relatively peaceful and predictable ending, which can be made more so with good pain management. Some people, however, suffer greatly at the end of life; in some cases they literally go out kicking and screaming, because they are suffering from either advanced delirium or pain that is difficult to control.

Medical assistance in dying, even years after legalization, is still an anomaly, accounting for fewer than 2 percent of deaths in Canada. Since the law took effect in February 2016 (December 2015 in Quebec), there have been fewer than fourteen thousand MAID deaths. Yet almost all those choosing a hastened death are elders; the average age is 75. One of the most challenging aspects of MAID, legally and ethically, is whether it should be available to patients with dementia. In other words, can someone determine, in advance, that they will want to end their life even if they will not be legally competent when the procedure is carried out?

More than anything else, the legalization of assisted death has forced us to have uncomfortable, and sometimes previously unthinkable, conversations about death. It has also empowered elders, giving them control over the penultimate moment in life.

Some of those choices have made for heart-wrenchingly beautiful endings, such as the story of George and Shirley Brickenden, aged 95 and 94 respectively, who opted to die together after almost seventy-three years of marriage. On March 27, 2018, the couple, who between them suffered an alphabet soup of health conditions that had made their lives painful and at times unbearable, died holding hands in their own bed in a Toronto retirement home. The night before, they had held a farewell dinner with family, where they reminisced about lives well lived, and the day of the MAID procedure they sipped champagne and nibbled on lobster hors d'oeuvres before lying down one last time.

"It couldn't have been a better way to go. Totally peaceful," their daughter Angela recalls. "It allowed them to bow out gracefully together, as they lived."

Part Two

NO MORE

CHAPTER 9

Aging in Place

The legendary urbanist Jane Jacobs was once asked where elders should live, and her terse reply was: "Everywhere." Jacobs vigorously promoted the idea that cities, and the places that house people (homes, apartments, co-ops, institutions), should be inclusive, fun and, most of all, adapted to the needs of residents, not the other way around. Jacobs also believed in the organic nature of communities, that those that functioned best were self-organized and a bit chaotic, not sterile and planned.

Janet Torge, a 73-year-old filmmaker from Montreal, believes that is exactly the philosophy we need to embrace as we reinvent eldercare. "It's painfully clear that we need better housing options, especially for seniors," she says. For years Torge has been promoting an approach she calls "Radical Resthomes," or "Houses with Purpose," multi-generational, freewheeling homes where people choose who they live with and set their own rules, "instead of being dumped all together with a bunch of strangers in a building that smells like piss."

Torge says she developed a passion for improving seniors' housing as she saw her parents and those of her friends end up living and dying unhappily in institutional care. Not only were she and her peers racked with guilt, they were determined they would not meet the same fate themselves. While Torge's mother died when she was young, her father spent his final years in a nursing home, which she describes as a prison for the incarcerated elderly. "He would say: 'I don't like it here, but that's the deal, that's what we do with old people.' But my generation is not going to stand for that. We want a new deal."

The Radical Resthomes concept is fairly simple, a mix of a co-op and a retirement home, with a couple of twists. Torge says the key is bringing together people, young and old, with similar interests or values—for example, a rest home for artists, or entrepreneurs or lesbians, or Serbian speakers. The elders would mentor the younger residents, who would in turn invigorate the elders' lives and stave off the loneliness that afflicts so many older people. "I don't know why policy-makers think old people only want to live with old people. We don't. We want to be active members of our community," Torge insists.

In the rest homes as envisaged, all six to ten residents would have a private room, but there would be common spaces, including the kitchen and living room. The facilities would be multigenerational and people would share the chores and expenses, in the style of a kibbutz. The rent would be affordable for young and old alike, roughly in line with market prices, and about half the cost of seniors' complexes. If residents needed additional care, like PSWs, it would come from the outside. "Most importantly, we would die in our own beds, not in an institution," Torge says.

The Radical Resthomes idea has been greeted with great enthusiasm, including by the Solutions Lab of Canada Mortgage and Housing Corporation, a program that funds innovative housing projects. The sticking point for Torge is that she wants to start small, build a prototype, then use the equity to build similar homes around the country. But this plan flies in the face of the more grandiose schemes government policy-makers tend to seek out: projects that require developers with millions of dollars.

"Everybody who has evaluated this idea loved it, but the catch is that it's almost too simple and easy. They want everything to be big. They can't get their minds beyond funding big towers because they think there's this tsunami of helpless old people coming," Torge explains. "What they don't seem to realize is that we aren't helpless, and we don't want to live in those damn towers." She is now working with private developers because they are far more willing to embrace innovative ideas.

Torge is right, of course. With all the talk of a silver tsunami, soaring health care costs, horrific mortality rates in nursing homes and other apocalyptic news about seniors, it is easy to forget that the vast majority of elders in Canada are happy and healthy and live independently. Research conducted by the Public Health Agency shows that about three in five Canadians described their health as good or excellent. Notably, the rates are highest in people under 19 and over 65, the youngest and oldest demographics. The challenge, for elders in particular, is to help them remain in that healthy, happy state for as long as possible, and the principal precondition for that remains living independently.

Currently, about 7 percent of Canadians over the age of 65 live in institutions such as long-term-care homes, nursing homes and hospitals. While that is among the highest rates in the world, it's also a reminder that 93 percent of elders live in the community, most in their own residences. The challenge, from a public policy perspective, is to maximize the time they spend there, aging in place, since the number of elders who live in the community drops sharply as people get older. Almost one-third of those over 85 live in nursing homes, as do more than half of centenarians.

Home care services have a role to play in helping people stay in their homes, but, in the grand scheme of things, it's just a tiny piece of the puzzle. If we want people to age in place, we need to ensure that the homes and cities they live in are senior-friendly. The homes where elders live need to be senior-proofed in the same way family homes are baby-proofed to keep children safe, for example by removing throw rugs and assessing other fall hazards in a dwelling.

We need to modify building codes so that features such as doorways wide enough for wheelchairs, ramps, and grab bars in tubs and showers become standard features instead of ones that require costly renovations. Municipalities, if they value seniors, need to prioritize services like sidewalk clearing, well-lit streets and public transport. Inclusivity needs to be built into public policies.

Being senior-friendly also means bringing services to people instead of making them travel. The main reason elders are driven out of their homes is not illness but everyday barriers to getting around in the community, such as insufficient public transportation and the lack of enough restrooms and elevators in public spaces. Combined with social factors such as isolation and unaffordable housing, aging in place can be impossible for many.

While the population is aging, it is not doing so in a uniform fashion. Elders increasingly live in clusters, in buildings or in neighbourhoods, a phenomenon academics call naturally occurring retirement communities (NORCs), which provide an opportunity to deliver services differently and allow people to remain in the community longer.

An example of a NORC is Oasis Senior Supportive Living in Kingston, Ontario. Most of the residents in the fifty-unit building had been living there for many years. Collectively, they weren't getting any younger; they would get a stark reminder of this when, every now and then, one of their neighbours would be carted off to a nursing home. So, about a decade ago, the residents, with the help of researchers at Queen's University, decided to create a system of on-site social supports. The guiding principle was that elders should remain self-sufficient for as long as possible and that it was in the interest of the public, private and not-for-profit sectors to work together to help make that a reality.

At Oasis, the landlord provides a space for communal activities—everything from bingo to exercise classes to making meals. A number of programs, paid for with government grants and charitable donations, were created to combat the scourges of aging, including loneliness, inactivity and malnutrition.

The Queen's professors, Catherine Donnelly and Vince DePaul, found that the simple interventions had an impact well beyond the building. Emergency room visits and hospitalizations for residents of the building fell noticeably, and those who were hospitalized had shorter stays compared with the period prior to the creation of Oasis. Demand for home care fell about 10 percent. Surveys of residents revealed that they were happier, healthier and less lonely than seniors in the community at large. The program also provides residents' family members with peace of mind. "They know that their mom or dad are being watched over," says Helen Cooper, chairperson of the Oasis board and a former Kingston mayor. The total cost of the program works out to a little less than $10 a week per resident.

NORC is a term coined in the early 1980s by Michael Hunt, professor of urban planning at the University of Wisconsin–Madison, who studied the makeup of apartment complexes in Madison. Because physical and social environments play an important role in determining the health of populations, he hypothesized that the communities where people were able to remain as they aged would be healthier than others. The theory was borne out by years of research, not only in apartment complexes but in mobile home parks, condos and neighbourhoods with family homes.

In his work, Professor Hunt was able to determine not only the characteristics of NORCs but the policy initiatives that could facilitate their creation and help elders age in place. NORCs were not necessarily clusters of wealthy people, but they always emerged in vibrant communities, where people were physically and socially active. Population density was always high, and regardless of the actual crime rate NORCs were perceived as safe and crime-free. Good public transit was another key characteristic, as were walkable streets, and stores within walking distance. Professor Hunt found that relatively basic policies such as keeping sidewalks clear of snow and extending the duration of walk signals so people had more time to cross intersections made an appreciable difference. While it may seem counterintuitive, the presence of bike paths and children's play facilities was also important, because healthy elders like to have their children and grandchildren around. Since many seniors do not drive, having neighbourhood shuttles in addition to good bus service helps them age in place.

Professor Hunt notes that NORCs exist principally in cities, which isn't surprising given that more than 80 percent of elders live in urban areas. Even those who lived most of their lives in rural areas tend to migrate to cities to be closer to services and family members.

While NORCs hold promise, they only exist, or can be created, in areas where people own or rent their homes. One of the biggest barriers to aging in place is lack of affordable housing, so seniors end up moving in with other family members or into institutions like long-term-care homes. Governments are far more likely to subsidize institutional care for elders than they are to subsidize their housing costs in the community, even if they are a fraction of the cost.

But there are some aging-in-place initiatives that combine low-cost housing and community care. One of them is SPRINT, Senior Peoples' Resources in North Toronto. The community group, founded in the early 1980s, oversees the care of residents in four Toronto Community Housing buildings; it also operates an innovative long-term-care facility for people with dementia and a transitional site for "alternate level of care" patients waiting for a permanent spot in care. "Most people know about long-term-care homes, but there are other, more attractive ways of living as you age, like assisted living or supportive housing," says Stacy Landau, CEO of SPRINT. (As in every other area of eldercare, there is a nomenclature issue: government uses the term "assisted living" while community groups prefer "supportive housing." Regardless of what you call it, the approach is to bring care to people in their homes, and subsidize rent and services so they are affordable.)

Supportive housing is a bit of a hybrid of home care and LTC. SPRINT provides a wide variety of services, including personal care, Meals on Wheels, transportation, respite care, and activities like knitting and baking. People live in their homes—in this case subsidized apartments—and staff work exclusively in SPRINT's buildings instead of doing contract work in people's homes. That allows a lot more flexibility in the delivery of care to residents, who range in age from 70 to 108.

"We do short episodes of care, which is what most people really want. Instead of two hours of care on a Tuesday afternoon, which is what people might get at home, we can provide fifteen minutes one morning, thirty minutes the next afternoon, and so on," Landau says. The staff ratios are 1:5 during the day and 1:10 at night, much better than in most long-term-care homes. Having permanent staff on-site means workers spend their time providing hands-on care, not travelling between locations as they do in community home care. There is also far less turnover, which allows continuity of care; some people have had the same support workers for twenty-five years.

Landau stresses that the community group cannot provide the same level of care as a long-term-care facility, but they can get creative to help people remain in their homes. For example, paramedics will visit to help with minor medical needs such as changing dressings or assessing injuries if someone falls. SPRINT also works closely with a group of geriatricians who do house calls.

As an example of the kind of medical attention residents receive, Landau recalls a home visit where a doctor came, along with a trainee, to check up on a patient who had recently been injured in a fall. Once in the apartment, the doctor noticed that a light bulb was burned out in the kitchen. He asked the student to find a sturdy chair and change the bulb, then told him: "That's probably the most effective thing we will do today, because it will likely prevent another injury."

Naheed Rahim, a PSW since 1996, explains SPRINT's philosophy of care: "We do what people need. When I leave a client, I feel good, and I want them to feel good." She sees eight to twelve clients in a day, for varying lengths of time depending on their needs. "Mr. Jones may want a shower, then I will remind him to take his medication, then I will go down the hall and give Mrs. Smith lunch, then go to another and make the bed and take out the garbage," she says.

Rahim observes that this is very different from working in the community, where you have one- or two-hour blocks of time and assigned tasks to carry out, whether the client wants them or not. An immigrant from Guyana, Rahim took a PSW course at George Brown College shortly after she arrived in Canada. Twenty-five years later, she says she has never considered changing jobs because the work is quite rewarding. "Personal care is so important for people's dignity and they get embarrassed when they can't do things themselves anymore, like take a shower. I help and they're very grateful."

She says that, above all, residents appreciate being able to stay in their own homes, and they often talk with dread about the alternative: long-term care. Because Rahim has worked in one place for so long, the clients also become like family. "When they pass, it's like losing a friend." She attends clients' funerals and was particularly touched when she was invited by a family to sit shiva.

Rahim says the work is also humbling, especially at her age (66). "We're all getting older. This work taught me that you have a better life if you stay at home."

SPRINT clients have their housing subsidized by the City of Toronto while their personal care is paid for by the provincial Ministry of Health (for those on the dementia floors, it's the Ministry of Long-Term Care). But other services, like Meals on Wheels and transportation to medical appointments, have to be paid out of pocket, and some social programs are underwritten by charitable groups.

"To be honest, the money question is very complicated and confusing. We're funded but not fully funded," Stacy Landau says. Funding can come (or not) from half a dozen different provincial ministries. Despite the bureaucratic burden, funding for the administration and operation of community groups themselves has been frozen for more than two decades, so they have become increasingly dependent on contributions from the United Way and other charitable donations, as well as volunteers.

The complexity exists at the individual level as well. "It's a bit all over the map what people pay for and what they don't pay for. It often doesn't make any sense," Landau admits. What is clear is that residents of the City of Toronto buildings receive personal care at no cost. But Landau says her biggest frustration is SPRINT's inability to expand its services beyond the community housing units. "Everyone in our buildings gets great care, but if they live literally across the street, they won't, they will pay or co-pay," she explains.

The City of Toronto, with a population of 3 million, has only eighty-three buildings with subsidized spots for seniors. There are about 12,500 elders benefiting from the low-cost apartments, while another 10,900 are waiting for a place. The wait list for affordable housing for seniors is a staggering ten years.

Landau says the public would be shocked if they had any idea how many elders are barely scraping by in the community, struggling to pay their rent. Some are homeowners whose property taxes have appreciated tremendously over the decades, but they can't afford to sell because they have nowhere to move. "There are a lot of women over 85 who are house poor or apartment poor; each month they have to choose between paying the rent or eating, and they can't go to retirement homes or long-term care because those aren't affordable either."

In the wake of Covid-19 and the shocking number of deaths in LTC, Landau's biggest fear is that governments will put all their attention and money into making those facilities safer and building more of them. That, she said, would be a disaster.

"We have to fundamentally rethink the challenge of caring for people as they age. We can't rethink long-term care in isolation," she insists. "We have to consider the place of community care, of supportive housing, of aging in place. There's nothing more important than where people live."

CHAPTER 10

Around the World

Ask virtually any expert where in the world is the best place to grow old and the answer, almost 100 percent of the time, will be Denmark.

It's not hard to see why.

The tiny Nordic country, population 5.8 million, started building its social welfare state almost a century ago, and today it has an enviable palette of cradle-to-grave social programs. Just as important, Danes believe that every citizen has a right to enjoy a meaningful and dignified life, regardless of age or economic means. That philosophy means that elders are not shunted out of sight and out of mind; rather, they are integrated into everyday life and expected to be active members of the community.

Denmark is a country where 90-year-olds really do ride around on bikes. Of course, some of its elders need care, and while the care on offer is extensive, the approach is to empower elders in caring for themselves. Again, this is diametrically opposed to what usually happens in Canada, where the structure of home care and long-term care leads to infantilizing, deconditioning and dependence.

One of the great advantages Denmark gave itself was heeding the warnings of demographers. Back in the early eighties, when the impact of the aging baby boom generation began to grow apparent and demographic nihilism became voguish, it was one of the few countries to start planning ahead. It did not dither, nor did it see an aging population as a catastrophe. Instead, Denmark took a deliberate decision to make healthy aging a priority, and this included rejecting institutionalization. Danish elders were not going to be confined to hospitals and nursing homes; they were going to stay in the community.

To this day, Denmark invests far more extensively in home care than almost any other country. There are even financial penalties imposed on municipalities if elders are deemed to be institutionalized unnecessarily. While the principal argument against going all-in on home care is that it costs too much, Denmark's example shows you get what you pay for: the country has only slightly more hospital and nursing home beds today than it had four decades ago. Unlike Canada, it does not have a single "alternate level of care" patient; patients are discharged from hospital promptly, either to a rehab facility, back to their home, or to a long-term-care facility. The nursing homes that do exist are reserved for the sickest of the sick. They are also quite modern and well staffed, because caring for elders is a societal priority.

The country's overall health spending is about middle of the pack among OECD nations. (And while Denmark's universal health care system is much more extensive than Canada's—including home care, LTC, prescription drugs, mental health care, rehab and more—it actually spends less per capita.)

Denmark, like Canada, has a decentralized health system. The federal government provides block grants from tax revenues to the regions and municipalities, which deliver health services. Regions own, manage and finance hospitals, as well as financing the large majority of services offered by health professionals, from physicians through to pharmacists and dentists. Municipalities are also responsible for most services used by elders, including home care, home help, nursing homes and rehabilitation.

One of the key elements of the Danish system is that general practitioners are responsible for medical follow-up of patients, regardless of whether care is delivered in clinics, in hospitals or at home. There are mandatory agreements between regions and municipalities to ensure care is coordinated. It is a long-standing policy that everyone should be able to live at home as long as possible, and there are funding incentives for everything from reducing hospital admissions to ensuring follow-up home visits.

Coordination initiatives between health and social welfare programs place an emphasis on people with complex health needs, most of whom are frail seniors. The focus of all eldercare programs is helping citizens maintain—or regain—autonomy, often through rehabilitation and re-ablement. For example, instead of cooking for a person with failing eyesight, an occupational therapist will work with them to adapt their cooking to their physical limitations. The underlying philosophy is to not do anything for people that they can do for themselves, to keep them as independent as possible. In that vein, technology plays a vital role. A widely used device is the "pill robot," which electronically reminds elders to take their medication and ensures the right dosage at the right time. Because Denmark has an electronic health record that is fully integrated across the health system, the robot is updated in real time if a physician or pharmacist changes a prescription.

There are, of course, elders who do need institutional care because they require 24/7 medical oversight, including patients with advanced dementia. But Danish nursing homes would be largely unrecognizable to Canadians, as they tend to be small, home-like facilities integrated into the community. When municipalities build new nursing homes, the priority is to ensure residents can have a safe, socially active life, and that staff will have a supportive work environment. Ceiling lifts, bathing chairs, and beds with patient-turning systems are all standard equipment. As a result, residents are kept more mobile and there are fewer broken hips and pressure ulcers, and staff suffer far fewer injuries. Care homes are considered to be living labs where new technologies are tested. Innovations include a wetness sensor to ensure incontinence pads are changed promptly; when the digital tool was tested, it ended up saving thirty-two minutes a day for care aides because fewer checks were required and there were fewer leaks that necessitated clothing changes.

While eldercare in Denmark is impressive, it is not perfect. Tensions exist between the federal, regional and municipal levels of government; there are worries about the ever-escalating cost of health and social services; and there are some who believe individuals should take more responsibility, financial and otherwise. Still, these challenges exist in every country and every jurisdiction.

We have to remember, too, that the way eldercare is funded and delivered is not just a medical or financial issue. Public policies are heavily influenced by a country's history, politics and values. No matter how enviable the Danish eldercare system may look from afar, trying to replicate it in Canada would likely fail. But we can learn from it, and adapt best practices to suit our particular needs.

There is a French proverb that says: *Quand on se regarde, on se désole; quand on se compare, on se console.* There is no pithy English equivalent, but it essentially means: "When we look at ourselves, we despair; when we compare ourselves to others, we take comfort."

One of the principal reasons to examine how other countries treat their elders is to learn from their successes and failures. So here is a brief overview of approaches in other countries—food for thought to allow us both to despair and to take comfort.

Australia

Australia is the country whose health system most closely resembles Canada's: its eldercare system is overly dependent on institutional care, wait lists are endless, and oversight is virtually non-existent. Australia also has a similar mix of private and public delivery, and funding that is at odds with its universal medicare system. A seemingly endless series of stories about abuse and neglect that were exposed by the media led to the creation of the Royal Commission into Aged Care Quality and Safety in 2019. In its interim report, the commission said bluntly that care is dismal: "We have found that the aged care system fails to meet the needs of our older, often very vulnerable, citizens. It does not deliver uniformly safe and quality care for older people. It is unkind and uncaring towards them. In too many instances, it simply neglects them." In response to the interim report, the federal government announced a significant increase in funding for home care services that will allow some patients to choose an alternative to institutional care. In 2021, however, the commission is expected to issue its final report that will propose a complete revamp of eldercare. Canadian politicians and policy-makers should pay close attention.

Brazil

In Brazil, LTC is provided in hospitals. About 2.5 percent of hospital beds are set aside for chronic patients, and the care is largely state-funded. In a country of 210 million, there are only about forty thousand elders receiving home care services.

China

In accordance with Chinese tradition, LTC is provided principally by family members at home. Care homes and home care are not covered by public health insurance. Because of the long-standing one-child policy and the growing mobility of younger citizens, an increasing number of elders do not have family support. They end up either in community hospitals or as paupers in makeshift facilities where the quality of care is dismal at best. A number of private providers have also sprung up, catering to middle-class and wealthy families. The government's stated goal is to create a national long-term insurance program but, to date, 60 million people are in pilot projects.

England

The National Health Service pays for home care and nursing home care for people whose medical needs arise from illness, disability or accident. About 135,000 people are eligible for this coverage. Other eldercare services are paid either out of pocket or by local health authorities, based on a needs test and a means test. In a country of 56 million, about 870,000 people receive long-term-care services either at home or in institutions—roughly the same proportion as in Canada. However, unlike in Canada, the large majority of eldercare, about 75 percent, is delivered in the home. England has what is widely considered the world's best end-of-life care; palliative care is offered in the home, in care homes and in hospices.

France

As in many countries, the provision of LTC in France cuts across a number of policy sectors—health care, social welfare, housing and seniors—and coordination is a challenge. So too is funding, which comes from three levels of government and a variety of programs. France has a very hospital-centric health system, and traditionally elders were cared for either by their family or in hospital. In a country of 68 million, there are more than 10,000 long-term-care homes (often extensions of hospitals) with 730,000 beds. All medical and care costs are covered, but families are responsible for the cost of accommodation. Home care is also medically oriented, provided principally by physicians and nurses. The development of a community sector is relatively recent. Elders with physical limitations, as well as people with disabilities, are entiled to an "autonomy allowance" to pay for services. It is funded by the National Solidarity Fund for Autonomy; one day a year, employees work for free and employers pay the forfeited wages into the fund.

Germany

In Germany, long-term-care insurance is mandatory, and provided by the same insurers who provide health insurance. Employees contribute 3.05 percent of their gross salary to fund Social Health Insurance. However, long-term-care benefits cover only about half the cost of institutional care. In a country of 83 million, about 3.4 million Germans have supplementary insurance. However, anyone with a physical or mental illness or a disability, regardless of age, can apply for additional benefits, which vary based on the level of care required. There is a separate program that pays family caregivers up to 50 percent of home care costs. Germany also has an extensive network of hospices and palliative care wards that are publicly funded.

India

India, with a population of 1.3 billion, is home to about 130 million elders. In theory, under the terms of the National Program for

Health Care for the Elderly, they all have access to "free, specialised health care facilities exclusively for elderly people" (everyone over age 60). The program, launched in 2011, was supposed to create geriatric units in at least a hundred hospitals, along with eight "super-facilities." However, in practice, LTC is virtually nonexistent. Public hospitals tend to be overcrowded and offer poor-quality care. About 75 percent of health care, including LTC, is privately funded in India and out of reach for many citizens, particularly in rural areas. Abandoning elders is still shockingly common, and they depend on charitable organizations for very basic food and shelter.

Japan

Japan has the world's oldest population and some of the world's most extensive eldercare. Traditionally, eldercare was the responsibility of families, and women in particular. But the aging of the population, combined with increased numbers of women in the workforce, meant that many elders ended up living in hospital. To address the costly problem of "social hospitalization," the federal government created a long-term-care insurance (LTCI) program in the year 2000. LTCI is compulsory, and funded by federal and municipal governments, as well as employers. It covers a broad range of services, including long-term-care facilities, home care, respite care, assistive devices and home modification. Elders make copayments of 10 to 20 percent of the cost of services. The most remarkable feature of the Japanese model is that it allows one-stop shopping. Elders undergo a thorough assessment, their care requirements are determined, and then they are allocated a budget; clients have a broad range of services and providers to choose from.

Netherlands

The Netherlands spends more per capita on eldercare than any other country. Coverage is universal and extensive—residential care, home care, personal care, nursing care, assistive devices and transportation services—but funded separately from the universal health care program. The Long-Term Care Act was created in 2015. The large majority of eldercare is provided in the home, chiefly by self-organized nursing units. Personal budgets are provided to patients, who organize and purchase their own care. In institutional care, patients pay accommodation costs.

Norway

In Norway, the majority of long-term-care recipients, about 70 percent, receive care at home; 20 percent live in nursing homes that provide 24/7 care; and 10 percent live in assisted housing facilities designed for elders. One in four home care patients have extensive needs that in most countries would require institutional care. Norway has virtually no private care providers. While the country has universal health care, which includes home care, institutional care is means-tested (meaning subsidies are available only to those below a certain income level), and cost-sharing can be high, with residents contributing anywhere from nothing to 85 percent of their income, depending on earnings. End-of-life care is provided in nursing homes; there are virtually no hospices. Family caregivers can apply for financial support and pension credits if they take time off work to care for loved ones.

Sweden

Sweden, like all Nordic countries, promotes home care over institutional care, with elders entitled to live at home as long as possible.

Only 28 percent of elders with long-term-care needs live in institutions. LTC is the responsibility of municipalities, which generally reimburse informal caregivers, either directly or by paying home care workers. Eligibility for services is based on need, but there is no means-testing.

United States

About 8.3 million people in the US require LTC, and one-third of them have extensive needs. That includes about 1.4 million living in nursing homes and 800,000 in residential care. There is no universal health care in the US, but Medicare covers most health care services for people over 65. However, LTC falls beyond the scope of Medicare. As a result, most LTC, whether institutional care or home care, is purchased privately. Those who cannot afford it can apply for Medicaid coverage. The Affordable Care Act (commonly known as Obamacare) included an ambitious plan to create a universal, voluntary, public long-term-care insurance program, but it was deemed unworkable and repealed. Long-term-care insurance is available but rarely purchased.

CHAPTER 11

Lest We Forget

Every year on November 10, hundreds of volunteers gather in an auditorium at Sunnybrook Health Sciences Centre in Toronto before heading outside to plant 47,500 Canadian flags on the lawn. When the 475 residents of the Sunnybrook Veterans Centre (SVC) awaken the next morning and put on their uniforms for Remembrance Day ceremonies, they are greeted by a sea of tiny Maple Leafs that resembles a field of poppies.

In Canadian society, few people garner more admiration and respect than veterans, especially the aging combat veterans of the Second World War and the Korean War. And respect is the bedrock of the care they receive at SVC, which is often referred to as the "Cadillac of long-term care" in Canada. "What we aim to achieve is the best life experience for every resident," says Dr. Jocelyn Charles, medical director of the Veterans Centre. "It's a mission we take seriously."

Sunnybrook Health Sciences, now one of Canada's largest hospitals and the country's premier trauma care facility, was originally built as a soldiers' hospital, solely for the care of veterans of the First and Second World Wars. (Prior to the advent of medicare, only veterans were entitled to "free" medical care.) At the inauguration in June 1948, Prime Minister William Lyon Mackenzie King said: "Sunnybrook Hospital symbolizes the sacrifices made by those members of the Armed Forces whom this hospital aims to serve and seeks to honour."

At its peak, Veterans Affairs Canada operated some forty facilities across Canada. As the demand for acute treatment and rehabilitative services decreased following the Korean War, the number of departmentally run facilities was reduced to eighteen by the mid-1950s, along with a shift in focus to the provision of mainly chronic care for veterans. Today, Veterans Affairs does not operate any facilities directly, but contracts "beds" in provincially run care homes around the country. The only two former military facilities that still cater exclusively to veterans are Sunnybrook Veterans Centre in Toronto and Ste. Anne's Hospital in Sainte-Anne-de-Bellevue, Quebec.

The average age of SVC residents is 96. There are as many centenarians as there are youngsters under the age of 100. Dementia is the norm among this battle-scarred cadre of elders, and they are handled with care; every effort is made to give the large facility a homelike feel. "This is not a long-term-care home that people dread coming to," Dr. Charles says. "Our facility is a destination they want to come to because they and their families know they're going to have a good life here."

That isn't empty boasting, and Janice Henty can attest to it. Her father, Jack Marshall, a Halifax bomber pilot in the Second World War, spent the last four years of his life living in the Veterans Centre before his death in July 2020 at age 96.

Henty knew very little about Sunnybrook before her father moved there, but the family had been eager to get him out of a retirement home where care was second-rate and the cost was exorbitant. "To be honest, initially, I wasn't impressed. The building isn't imposing at all. It's old and it looks like a hospital," she recalls.

"But my attitude changed the minute I saw how Dad was treated." A long-time professor of nursing at George Brown College in Toronto, Henty says she was immediately struck by both the professionalism and the empathy of the staff, from the janitors through to the nurses, and over the years her admiration would only grow. "As part of my work I've visited many, many nursing homes, and I've never seen anything where the quality of care compares to Sunnybrook."

Combat veterans, unlike most Canadian elders, have ready access not only to top-notch institutional care but to extensive home care, both of which are heavily subsidized by Veterans Affairs Canada. The goal of its Veterans Independence Program (VIP) is to ensure aging veterans remain healthy and independent in their principal residence—be it a family home, an apartment or a seniors' home—as long as possible; and when they can no longer live at home, they will get institutional care. And because both are affordable, they actually have a choice.

The home care services that VIPs are entitled to are far more extensive than those conferred upon civilians. The services include not only nursing care (without the daily caps set by provinces) but wound care, occupational therapy and rehabilitation services. Personal care by PSWs is also supplied, but so too is housekeeping and grounds maintenance, such as cutting the lawn. VIPs also receive nutritional support, which means that a service like Meals on Wheels, which most elders pay out of pocket, would be supplied free of charge.

Jack Marshall was healthy and active well into his 80s—he suffered from some heart problems and hearing loss—so he used few of the VIP benefits available to him. He and his wife, Audrey, moved out of the family home in 2008 and into a condo, so he didn't need to access the maintenance services, but he did get help with housekeeping and home care services on top of those he received from the province, along with hearing aids at no cost. After Audrey died in 2012, he remained in the condo but began to suffer from cognitive issues, and was eventually diagnosed with Lewy body dementia.

In August 2015, Jack moved to a retirement home, Sunrise Senior Living, where his health took a turn for the worse. He lost fourteen pounds in two months, and then caught pneumonia. As his care needs increased, so did the bill. Unlike long-term-care homes, retirement homes charge extra for nursing care and PSWs. Jack's monthly bill was initially $4,000 but quickly jumped to more than $7,000.

Henty says her father was unhappy in the retirement home but also a bit reluctant to move to a long-term-care home, in part because Audrey had not had a good experience in that setting. She had moved to a municipally owned home in Toronto, but basic services such as bathing and toileting were so inadequate that the family hired a full-time, forty-hour-a-week PSW to take care of her. In total, her care ended up costing $9,600 a month. "Dad was a chartered accountant. He did well saving his money, so he could afford it. But we were not at all happy with the care," Henty says.

If eligible veterans choose to go into LTC, that is also subsidized. They pay only accommodation costs, not for any care. When Jack moved to Sunnybrook Veterans Centre in January 2016, his monthly fee was $980. (Over the next four years that would increase slightly to $1,058.) By comparison, the provincially regulated rate for a semi-private room in Ontario is $2,280 monthly. "Quite the difference," his daughter notes. "But money isn't what matters the most." SVC, she says, is the gold standard of eldercare.

This is not to suggest it is perfect. Back in 2013, the Canadian Press published a series of articles calling into question the quality of care there, which prompted the federal government to order an audit. The complaints included unexplained injuries, rough

treatment, neglect of basic hygiene and infection control procedures, delayed feedings, residents abandoned for hours on end or
left languishing in bed for days, and a dearth of physiotherapy or
rehabilitation opportunities. That damning media coverage was a
catalyst to turn things around. In the wake of that audit, regular
provincial inspections were put in place, the complaints process
was changed, and internal structures were modified to ensure families had more of a voice in setting policies.

While the building is indeed not much to look at, several
wings have been added to the Veterans Centre over the years, and
they are divided into intimate units with thirty to forty residents,
each with dedicated staff. One of those units is Dorothy Macham
Home, a special ten-bed unit for veterans with severe behavioural
issues that was built in 2001. Most of the residents there have severe
dementia and war-related post-traumatic stress disorder and,
because of their illness, can be violent or highly disruptive. Everything is done to create a soothing environment and to try to understand the sources of their suffering. "Behaviours mean unmet
needs, so we figure out what those needs are," Dr. Charles says.
Again, the approach here is markedly different from most long-term-
care homes, where disruptive residents are routinely expelled and
tend to end up in locked psychiatric wards.

The resident-to-nurse ratio in the Veterans Centre is 5:1, a standard that is unheard of in the community. The majority of public
and private long-term-care facilities don't even have ratios of 5:1
for PSWs, never mind nurses. But at SVC, there are no PSWs. All
the work, even the personal care, is done by registered practical
nurses and registered nurses. Dr. Charles, who started her career
as a PSW and became a nurse and then a physician, says that isn't
a knock on PSWs but rather a deliberate decision to ensure the
best possible care for veterans who have complex health needs.

"Our nurses are all trained on how to spot a change in health status. They give standardized reports to physicians so we can intervene quickly when any medical issue arises."

The SVC also boasts an impressive cadre of support staff, including music therapists, horticultural therapists, audiologists, pharmacists, opticians, chaplains, art therapists, physiotherapists, occupational therapists, foot care technicians and more. Dr. Charles says these services are not just nice to have but essential. While traditional care focuses on achieving the best clinical outcomes using accepted scientific evidence and traditional practice methods, Sunnybrook embraces a care philosophy known as ABLE (achieving best life experience).

Unlike in many nursing homes, veterans eat and sleep when they want. Recreational activities are also tailored to their interests. There is live music three times a week in the home's stunning foyer, known as the Warrior's Hall. There are also daily outings to shopping malls, sporting events, theatres and legion halls—activities that are sponsored by the Royal Canadian Legion. Residents also have a pub, a barber shop and a branch of the Toronto Public Library on site, as well as access to a beautiful garden. Dr. Charles likes to tell the story of one resident with dementia who made it a habit to uproot the flowers in the garden. When the landscaper complained, the nurse caring for the man replied: "But it's his garden."

The medical director says the mantras that guide care at SVC are "anticipate unmet needs"—physical, social, emotional or based on past experience—and "go with the flow." If residents are safe and happy, that's what matters most.

The big question, of course, is whether the level of care afforded to respected veterans could be offered to all Canadian elders. Henty says that, sadly, she doesn't think so. "It costs a lot of money to provide this level of care. I'm not sure governments are willing do so."

The irony for her is that, while her father was a veteran, the war experience was not an important part of his life, and he had nothing to do with Veterans Affairs until the final years of his life, when he received a lot of extra care almost by happenstance.

But Dr. Charles has no doubt that the system created for veterans can and should be the norm, not the exception. "We have a good model and there's no reason it can't be duplicated for civilians," she insists. She acknowledges it would cost more money to offer people real choice between home care and LTC, and to make the choices affordable, but we shouldn't be nickel-and-diming elders just because they didn't go to war. The key, Dr. Charles says, is, first, making sure only those who really need institutional care end up there and, second, providing respectful care. "If a person has to go to long-term care, they should have expectations and those expectations should be met. We have to value everyone, not just veterans."

CHAPTER 12

A Prescription for Reform

If there is one thing Canada does better than any other country in the world, it is producing reports and recommendations on how to reform its health system. Since the advent of medicare, there have been at least 150 inquiries, parliamentary hearings, task forces and commissioned reports on the sad state of long-term care, home care and eldercare, not to mention media exposés, academic work and *cris de coeur* from families. And yet very few of the recommendations ever get implemented. The result is neglect by institutional indifference (a combination of bureaucratic inertia, constant political changing of the guard and fear of change), for which elders have paid a heavy price, before and during the pandemic.

We knew what reforms were needed before Covid-19 struck and now we know what needs to be done even more urgently. The most pointed message to take from the carnage wrought by the pandemic is that we need to stop wringing our hands and start implementing reforms in earnest. As one of the most recent reports—*Ageing Well* by the Covid-19 Health Policy Working Group of Queen's University—concluded: "The best time to change course and address the wellbeing of seniors was many years ago. The second-best time is right now."

We don't need any more sprawling judicial inquiries that produce weighty tomes to be shelved and forgotten. If there are to be more blue-ribbon committees, they must be given very specific tasks (for example, determine the minimum staffing levels required in long-term-care homes) and be required to provide detailed timetables and costing for the implementation of their recommendations.

Even more important, before any government appoints another expert group, they must commit up front to follow through—not ponder earnestly or cherry-pick, but implement fully. Reasonably, this should be done within a set budget; for example, a province could allocate $1 billion to upgrade the infrastructure of long-term-care homes and an expert committee could determine how to get the most bang for the buck. Unless we take this approach, we will simply end up with more reports serving as doorstops rather than blueprints for reform.

There are few things more disheartening than going back and reading old reports. One can't help but be struck by how the same problems are exposed and the same solutions are suggested, time and time again. The sombre takeaway is a sense that so much needs to be done that it feels as though the twelve labours of Hercules await us. But we also need a monumental shift in our approach. We have to ask ourselves fundamental questions such as, What do we want our lives to look like when we get old?

Of course, once you make such a philosophical commitment, much nuts-and-bolts work remains to be done. The fixes can't all be implemented at once, so we need to prioritize and pick our battles. What follows is a brief overview of the main areas that need to be addressed. This is not meant to be an exhaustive list of recommendations, but rather a broad prescription for how to improve eldercare. It is up to our political leaders and policy-makers to give life to these priorities and it is up to us, as citizens, to demand they do so.

So where should we start? Ideally, where the biggest problems exist.

Staffing

Health care is a people business—trained workers providing skilled care for patients in need. Yet Canada does not have a health human resources strategy. The type and number of health workers we have is based on long-ingrained practices more than anything else. Sadly, eldercare's roots in the penal system are still showing.

More than anything, the pandemic exposed how important front-line workers are, especially to frail elders; chronic labour shortages are as deadly as viruses. Covid-19 also graphically under-scored that the conditions of work are the conditions of care. Improving eldercare begins with fixing the work environment for nurses, PSWs and others. Staff need resources, structures, support and time to deliver quality care.

How many additional workers do we need? A lot. But deter-mining the proper staffing levels shouldn't be a guessing game. We need to guarantee patients a minimal level of care—for example, four hours daily of hands-on care in nursing homes. Then we need to provide funding. Making vague promises about funding four hours of care and then providing budgets that barely allow for three hours (as all provinces do) is simply embedding inadequate care into the system.

The mix of staff matters too. The workforce has not evolved to align with the increasingly complex health needs of elders. Quite the opposite, in fact. We need to get nurses back into nursing homes. The Registered Nurses' Association of Ontario has recommended that 20 percent of care be delivered by registered nurses, 25 percent by registered practical nurses and 55 percent by PSWs. Is that the ideal mix? Maybe, maybe not. But it's a good starting point for discussing the regulation of staffing ratios.

The complexity of patients in nursing homes (and home care, to a certain degree) also requires more involvement from physicians. The current approach, where much medical care is provided principally by retired doctors working part-time, is clearly inadequate. Residents shouldn't be shipped off to hospital emergency rooms every time they have a minor ailment, nor should they be getting care by fax. Much more medical care, up to and including palliative care, needs to be provided on-site, in facilities and homes.

We also need to ensure that all health care providers work to their full scope of practice and do the work they're trained to do, which will ensure their jobs are rewarding and that we get value for money.

Currently, about 80 percent of shifts in care homes and home care are not fully staffed, which creates an untenable situation. Addressing the shortage will take time and money. Nationally, only Quebec has committed to hiring ten thousand additional PSWs and to giving them full-time work with a living wage. That's a start. But we have to be careful of unintended (or unthought-of) consequences. Raising the wages of workers in LTC has decimated the home care workforce. Plundering one sector to bolster another is not a solution. The bottom line: we need national staffing standards—a care guarantee—and monitoring to ensure the regulations are respected.

Workers who do the valuable, sometimes back-breaking work that is eldercare should be paid a decent living wage. Full-time jobs with benefits should be the norm, not the exception. Health care workers, whether they are nurses, PSWs or food services workers, should be paid comparable wages regardless of where they work, be it a hospital, a care home or the community. (Currently, wages can be as much as $10 an hour less for those who work in the community.) A one-workplace policy should also be in place; workers juggling shifts at several facilities is bad for infection control—especially, but not exclusively, during a pandemic—and for continuity of care.

We cannot ignore that a large number of our care workforce are immigrants. We need to change immigration policies to favour those who are willing to work in eldercare, not just child care (nannies). At the height of the Covid-19 crisis, asylum seekers came to the rescue of long-term-care homes, particularly in Quebec, where they earned the moniker "guardian angels." Caring for our most vulnerable citizens should be a fast track to citizenship. Along the way, we need to reimagine geriatric care as a rewarding career, where workers are valued and respected.

As was stated in *Restoring Trust*, a report commissioned by the Royal Society of Canada: "If we do nothing else right now, we must solve the workforce crisis. It is *the* pivotal challenge."

Caregivers

While paid health care workers are essential, the vast majority of eldercare is provided by unpaid family and friends. Canadians of all ages offer this care willingly and lovingly. But caring for an aging spouse, parent or grandparent should not be driving people to an early grave. For the most part, families—which almost always means wives, daughters and granddaughters—provide care for loved ones at home until they burn out. Caregiving imposes steep costs on women's health, their family lives and their careers. That's not the way the "care journey" (to use a bit of a hackneyed term) should unfold. "We need to allow families to be families. We need to provide supports," says Tamara Daly, a political economist and health services researcher at York University.

Supports for caregivers can come in many forms. First and foremost, they need financial supports. Caregivers who take time off work need compensation similar to Employment Insurance. The programs that exist now are too rigid—time off is allowed only in the last months of a loved one's life. But the reality is that care needs come and go, and are not exclusive to end of life. Caregivers also need tax credits to offset their spending, which can be considerable. Tax deductions are not much use if you have little or no income because you have made a commitment to care for a family member.

Most of all, caregivers need to be offered real choice in their care options. Self-directed care programs are great in theory, but the bureaucracy is stultifying. People really want to help care for loved ones, but we have to make it easier.

"There are two knee-jerk reactions I hear over and over again: it's too expensive and people will abuse the system. The reality is people will ask for what they need, if that, with few exceptions," says Jennifer Baumbusch, an associate professor at the School of Nursing, University of British Columbia. "We have abused caregivers for a long time," she adds. "Isn't it time we offered them support, and respect?"

Long-Term-Care Homes

The worst thing that could happen in response to the Covid-19 pandemic is that we simply add more long-term-care beds by expanding current large facilities or building new ones. We don't need more warehousing of elders, or more inadequate care. We need better care.

For many high-needs patients, a nursing home is a good choice—or at least it should be. But placing elders in long-term-care facilities should not be the default setting; nor should it be a substitute for underfunded home care, or lack of access to affordable housing. The starting point for clearing the abominably long wait lists is ensuring that only those who need to be in LTC are the ones waiting for a bed.

While the quantity of care provided matters, we need to focus a lot more on quality of life in an institutional setting. Staffing, as already noted, is key. But the living environment matters too. Many nursing homes are old and not designed for the needs of today's residents. Their long, narrow hallways—dubbed "horridors"—don't accommodate wheelchair users, there's little access to the outdoors, and dining halls have more in common with prisons than homes.

After decades of duct tape solutions, Canada's provinces need to make judicious use of the wrecking ball. What needs to replace many of our large, decrepit institutions are smaller, more home-like facilities that are built to the needs of residents. For example, elders with dementia need to be able to wander safely, not just be confined to rooms; homes need to be equipped on the assumption that everyone could have mobility issues, with lifts to facilitate transfers from beds to walkers, and showers that are easily accessible to those who use walkers or wheelchairs.

Dragging the infrastructure and architecture into the twenty-first century won't happen quickly, and it won't be cheap, but it is essential. In the interim, we can reorganize to make existing facilities more user-friendly; with some effort, we can still provide pretty good care in big old buildings. The starting point is smaller units of care; even our current standard of 32-bed units is too impersonal. Small changes like cooking food on-site rather than microwaving prepackaged airplane-like meals make a big difference in quality of life.

As we upgrade and replace long-term-care homes, the following elements must all become standard: private or semi-private rooms and bathrooms, homey communal spaces, ready access to the outdoors, air conditioning, non-slip floors, laundry and cleaning services, and in-house food. As well, nursing homes should be an integral part of the community, not hidden away.

Home Care

Nobody knows exactly how many of the elders currently living in long-term-care facilities could be cared for at home; estimates vary from 20 to 50 percent. What is clear is that, in Canada, home care is grossly underutilized and underfunded. For every $1 spent on home care, $6 is spent on institutional care, which is one of the most imbalanced resource allocations in the developed world.

Aging at home is far and away the preference of elders, and if we want it to be a viable option, it has to be a deliberate policy choice, not an afterthought. Denmark, and a few other countries, have demonstrated that this approach is not only possible but preferable. Once there is a political commitment, implementation becomes a technical issue to be resolved. The non-system we have now would have to be revamped. As Shirlee Sharkey, CEO of the century-old home care provider SE Health, puts it: "No more tinkering. The system needs to be turned on its head."

The main problem with state-funded home care as it exists now is that it is managed like a task-based assembly line. Patients are allocated a set number of hours for specific tasks to be completed, whether they want them or not. Elders need choice and they need care to be personalized. The starting point has to be giving patients more choice, because, as stated earlier, people will request the help they truly need, with few exceptions.

The main hesitation about making home care the primary means of delivering eldercare arises from the notion that it would be too costly. The evidence, in academic research and in the experience of other countries, is that this is not true. And even if it were, so what? Gravel is cheaper than asphalt, but we wouldn't contemplate having dirt roads instead of paved roads.

One of the principal reasons home care is costly is that it is excessively bureaucratic, with one-third of dollars currently going to assessment. Money is better spent on actual care than on paying bureaucrats to limit access to that care. Elders and their family need to know up front what services are covered publicly and how much care they are entitled to.

Of course, there are limits, practical and financial, on what care can be provided in the home. What several European jurisdictions do is allow people to remain at home at least until their care costs exceed the cost of LTC. In Ontario, the province pays $180 daily for each person in long-term-care services. That money could go a long way towards keeping people where they want to be—at home—especially if they are allowed to use the funding creatively.

With a lot of pressure to expand home care in the wake of the pandemic, we have to be careful, however, to not simply shift the regimented, prescriptive rules imposed on elders from nursing homes to their own homes. Good home care is not just about avoidance of institutional care; it should provide more freedom and better quality of life.

Palliative Care

Being in care means your health is failing. Every elder, whether they are being cared for in hospital, in long-term care or at home, is sooner or later going to die.

While ensuring quality of life is paramount, that philosophy must extend to ensuring quality of death.

Planning for death has to be an integral part of every care plan, not last-minute improvisation. No elder should be dying without proper access to palliative care, whether they spend their final days in hospital, hospice, a nursing home or their own home.

Funding

"Current funding is insufficient to provide safe and dignified care," says Janice Legere, medical director at John Noble Home in Brantford, Ontario. That's the blunt truth: there is no question that money will be needed to fix what ails eldercare. There is a price to be paid for decades of neglect. With a bright light shone on the short-comings of institutional care during the coronavirus pandemic, there probably hasn't been a better time to invest, at least politically.

Governments across the country stepped up and spent hundreds of billions of dollars on Covid-19 relief programs. Relatively speaking, more will have been spent on the pandemic response than was spent on rebuilding the economy after the Second World War. In the grand scheme of things, the money needed to ensure better care for our elders represents little more than a rounding error.

Just as important as how much we spend, however, is *how* we spend. Currently, public health care funding is about $160 billion a year, $82 billion of which is spent on Canadians over the age of 65. So while we are already spending a lot on sickness care for elders, we are downright parsimonious when it comes to keeping them healthy in the first place: less than 5 percent of the health budget goes to prevention. A little more investment in rehab, re-ablement, and ensuring people are housed and fed could go a long way towards keeping elders out of institutional care.

Many Canadians assume that medicare will take care of them as they age. Sadly, that's not true. Unlike hospital and physician care—which are covered 100 percent under medicare—much elder-care requires private insurance and considerable out-of-pocket spending. People are denied essential care due to an inability to pay, which offends the principle of medicare and, frankly, feels un-Canadian. "With long-term-care facilities on the front lines of the Covid-19 crisis, the importance of universal, publicly funded, accessible health services has never been clearer," says Pat Armstrong, distinguished research professor of sociology at York University.

So how do you make eldercare universal and affordable?

There is much wonkish debate about whether or not the Canada Health Act should be amended to deem long-term care and/or home care "medically necessary" services. Politically, reopening the CHA would be a Pandora's box. It would be preferable to create a separate funding envelope in addition to the Canada Health Transfer, with monies targeted specifically for eldercare. It is essential that new funding come with clear strings attached. To be eligible for this federal funding, provinces would have to meet certain standards, such as staffing ratios.

In Canada, discussions about bolstering spending tend to focus on who will pay, individually and collectively. Private, for-profit nursing homes had some of the most deadly outbreaks during Covid-19, and the situation led to calls to ban for-profit facilities. But that solution is far from simple to implement, since up to 40 percent of nursing homes are for-profit in some provinces; simply banning them overnight would be catastrophic. Neither should it be assumed that not-for-profit facilities are magically safer or that they offer better care.

Private, for-profit homes exist, in large part, because governments are reluctant to spend on infrastructure. We have to remember also that all nursing homes—regardless of whether they are for-profit, not-for-profit or state-owned—receive the same (inadequate) stipend for care. If we regulate staffing ratios, that would largely eliminate the cutting of corners on labour costs. All nursing homes make their profits (or surpluses) by offering extra amenities; that would not change by deeming LTC a "medically necessary" service, nor would it eliminate people having to pay for the accommodation costs. In contrast to the different types of nursing homes, of much greater concern are for-profit retirement homes, which sell services, including essential care, à la carte, with little regulatory oversight.

Health care is a provincial responsibility, but the federal government has an important role in funding. Ottawa currently transfers about $40 billion to the provinces annually, a little more than 20 percent of total public spending. The feds need to contribute more, and eldercare is a perfect area in which to invest because it has national relevance.

For those arguing that we simply cannot afford to spend more, let's not forget that the non-system we have now is already costly, and inefficient to boot. As Michael Nicin of the National Institute on Ageing says: "It was going to be expensive to maintain a bad system. It will cost more to fix it. How much more? Who knows?"

Simply pumping more money into a broken system will achieve little more than to further ingrain mediocrity. As we reform eldercare, we need to focus on getting value for money. When we devalue eldercare, we devalue our elders.

Structure

Eldercare is a strange amalgam of long-term care, home care, seniors' housing and other social programs. There is no overarching system, and no one is in charge. The ministries responsible for caring for seniors operate, at best, in splendid isolation, and oftentimes at cross purposes.

A family with a loved one who has limited income and is struggling with dementia could easily find themselves trying to access half a dozen health and social programs under four different provincial ministries administered by a health region, a municipality and a couple of community groups, not to mention federal housing and income support programs.

At the very least, LTC, home care, retirement homes, assisted living and supportive housing should all be under the same provincial ministry, one whose ultimate goal should be to ensure that every elder is housed and cared for appropriately. "The fundamental problem we have is that we don't have a solid structure," says Miranda Ferrier, president of the Canadian Support Workers Association. "We have age-old problems with band-aid solutions. The pandemic came along and the band-aids fell off."

As much as politicians love cutting ribbons on new buildings, their constituents would be much better served by having services available in the community. The priority should not be building beds by expanding current facilities or constructing new ones, but serving individuals by giving them more choice about where and how they want to live.

Donna Duncan, CEO of the Ontario Long Term Care Association, likens the administration of eldercare in Canada to a game of Jenga, where players take turns removing one block at a time from a tower constructed of fifty-four blocks, then placing it on top, creating a progressively more unstable structure. "We have a system that has evolved over fifty years," she says. "We've added blocks, we've removed blocks, all without any real plan, and what we're left with is a fundamentally destabilized system."

We may not have built our eldercare in a considered manner, but now we have an unprecedented opportunity to create a system that stands on solid ground.

Regulation

Frail elders, especially those with dementia, are among the most vulnerable people in society. We need a good regulatory regime to ensure their protection. In the wake of the Covid-19 debacle, it has been suggested that what Canada needs are national standards, and perhaps that is true. But trying to create these standards would spark such a jurisdictional dispute that it would likely be more of a distraction from real reform than anything else.

In Canada's LTC and home care sectors, there is no lack of regulations, rules, norms and standards already. What's needed are not more rules, but smarter regulation. No one can seriously look back at the thousands of deaths that happened in long-term-care facilities during the pandemic and say: "None of this would have happened if only we had more bureaucracy."

The countries with the best eldercare—the same ones who have weathered Covid-19 well—also have the fewest regulations. Why? Because they have adequate staffing and funding. Models of care based on completing as many tasks or procedures as possible in a shift and ticking all the boxes are not how you deliver quality care. We need to move away from regulating the number of scoops of powdered mashed potatoes each resident receives if we want to make progress.

Of course, inspections are important, but they need to be done in a coherent, systematic fashion, and inspectors' reports have to be made public and easy to find and consult. A complaints-based process is not good enough. Nor are cursory visits every couple of years, only between the hours of nine and five.

Most of all, we need to change what we regulate, measure and reward. If a home can pass a fire inspection with flying colours even though it doesn't have a sprinkler system—because in some jurisdictions they are not mandatory—that does not mean residents are safe. Similarly, there's a need to standardize the recording of data such as the average number of falls in a home, since ten people falling in a month is very different from one person falling ten times. And the way we regulate can create perverse disincentives. For example, far too many people in nursing homes end up in wheelchairs because it's a way of minimizing falls; but being immobile is far worse for residents' health.

The data we collect tend to be a proxy for quality, not a measure of quality. Ultimately, what matters is the quality of care, not whether butter is stored at the proper temperature.

Advocacy/Information

When you speak to elders, their caregivers and care providers, there is one issue that comes up repeatedly and almost universally: how difficult it is to get basic information on accessing care. "The entry point to the system is unclear, the procedures to get care are complex, and the delays are much too long," says Eve-Lyne Couturier, a researcher at L'Institut de recherche et d'informations socioéconomiques (IRIS) in Montreal. "It's not normal that you need a GPS to find what services are available."

Elders and their families need to have an easy way of knowing what programs and services exist, and how to access them. Data must be publicly available so families can make informed choices. There needs to be a one-stop shopping portal, where the availability and cost of care are clearly articulated. Choice is important, and so is continuity of care. The needs of elders are varied and many, and they change over time; a cookie-cutter approach does not serve anyone well. "The health of older people is not static, so the care available to them should not be static," says Jennifer Baumbusch of UBC. We should be encouraging self-directed care options; but the programs themselves need to be far less bureaucratic in order to be user-friendly.

The patients with the most complex needs, such as those with dementia, require a navigator—a health professional such as a nurse who has an intimate knowledge of available services and how to access them—as a way of ensuring elders get the right care. (Nurse-navigators are common in cancer care; they are just as necessary in eldercare.) Canada has an excellent dementia strategy—at least on paper—but it has to be given life with funding and political commitment.

The pandemic, among other things, exposed the fact that elders don't really have a voice, especially those in institutional care. Tens of thousands of people were placed in lockdown for months, ostensibly to protect them from infection. These sorts of draconian measures should never have been imposed without residents and families having a say. Advocacy groups fought these restrictions, but, as outsiders, they had limited power. Residents' councils and family councils need to be empowered so their recommendations are implemented by managers and owners. Care homes are supposed to be *homes*, not prisons.

Every province should have a seniors advocate, an ombudsperson specifically for elders, as British Columbia has. During her tenure in that position, Isobel Mackenzie has done as much to improve eldercare as anyone in the country. We need more people with her passion to have the resources and power to hold governments' feet to the fire.

Community

Long-term-care homes and home care need a lot of attention. But we should not forget that the vast majority of elders live in the community, and our public policies should make that a priority. We need to stop with the elder apartheid and integrate care homes into the community. Facilities should be shared with daycares and schools. Being around older people, including people with dementia, should be a daily part of living, not an uncomfortable anomaly.

Building institutional beds is extremely costly. Affordable housing combined with home care services is far more cost-effective, and more humane. Having decade-long wait lists for supportive housing is a failure that needs to be corrected.

The only thing that keeps the disjointed, underfunded eldercare system from collapsing completely is the community sector, the thousands of community groups and volunteers, from Meals on Wheels to dementia advocates, who constantly find creative solutions to plug the gaps. A lot of the money going to bloated bureaucracies in health ministries and regional health authorities should be flowing directly to front-line community organizations.

In response to the global Covid-19 pandemic, we have taken a "Manhattan Project" approach. No effort has been spared, from unprecedented lockdowns, to billions of dollars in financial aid, to an all-hands-on-deck commitment to finding a coronavirus vaccine. Over a period of just months, society changed in ways that were previously unthinkable. Politicians acted with a boldness and forcefulness that is unheard of in peacetime. The level of social solidarity was inspiring.

We need to unleash a similar all-out effort to improve the care of elders. As we rebuild society and the economy, we have an opportunity to do things differently, to do them better. Elders have borne the brunt of the Covid-19 pandemic, and they should be the greatest beneficiaries as we come out the other side. "We need to create an environment where seniors can thrive, not just survive," says Jennifer Whiteside, secretary, business manager and chief spokesperson of the BC Hospital Employees' Union.

Ultimately, fixing eldercare is not about writing more reports, building more beds, spending more money or adopting new standards. It's about giving life to our values. If we love and value our parents, grandparents and great-grandparents—and, across the political spectrum, there is no question we do—then that must be reflected in our public policies.

It's long past time for the neglect to end.

Acknowledgements

In late April 2020, Anne Collins of Random House Canada sent me a short e-mail with the subject line "Long term care homes: is there a book to be done?"

An astute publisher, she wasn't interested in another book about Covid-19—of which there will be dozens—but rather a deep dive into one of the most glaring failures the pandemic exposed, Canada's inability (or perhaps unwillingness is a better word) to care properly for its elders. And she wanted it done quickly, while the issue was still top of mind.

As the health columnist at the *Globe and Mail*, the pandemic was already keeping me quite busy. In addition to writing columns for the paper, I was answering reader questions on various platforms including the Globe website, Facebook Live and Instagram, as well as making regular appearances on CBC's flagship radio program *The Current*. I also spend far too much time in Twitter. Such is a journalist's life in our multimedia world.

Taking on a quickie book project on top of this was perhaps not the wisest idea. But I was determined to find the time—early mornings, evenings, weekends and all my summer holidays— because I'm passionate about the issue for professional reasons and personal ones.

Both my parents experienced the cascade of care that is the fate of so many seniors as they age, chronic illness (Lewy body dementia for my dad; chronic obstructive pulmonary disease and vascular dementia for my mom), endless acute care and emergency room visits, selling the house to move into a seniors' residence, the health crises that trigger the need for long-term care, the seemingly unavoidable moves from one nursing home to another, and the painful declines in health and cognition leading to death.

Their care was frustratingly difficult to access, disjointed, costly and, ultimately, mediocre at best. In other words, typical. My father, who lived many years with dementia, died of an infection caused by a pressure ulcer (bedsore), which is indicative of neglect. My mom—all five foot nothing and ninety pounds of her—was kicked out of a couple of nursing homes for being "violent." It's not at all unusual for elders with dementia to lash out when they are frightened, and behaviours like slapping caregivers are cries for help more than anything. As a result, she lived her final months in an almost abandoned psychiatric hospital. The care there was actually great, but it was a sad, lonely existence; for people of my mom's generation, there is a lot of stigma about mental illness, and nobody wanted to visit her in the OH. (People of a certain age will recognize that shorthand for Ontario Hospital.)

The saving grace for my parents was that my brother, Marc, lived in the same city, and was an exceptionally generous and gifted caregiver. No one can survive our flawed eldercare system without an advocate at their side almost 24/7, and his relentless attention made our parents' lives better. Still, they deserved more from Canada's beloved medicare system. We all do.

All to say, the shortcomings of home care, LTC and the care of elders more generally have long rankled me. I have written often in my *Globe and Mail* columns about aging and its perils, in countless permutations. There are times when I can barely contain my fury at the indignities that continue to be endured by elders. That is equally true of my readers, who provide a great deal of feedback. The most passionate and desperate pleas for help always come from caregivers at the end of their rope struggling to understand how long-term-care homes and home care agencies have failed them so profoundly. Being able to examine those issues in more depth, in a book, was an opportunity I didn't want to pass up.

If what I have written is even semi-coherent, it is because I was blessed to have Pamela Murray, one of Canada's finest editors, oversee the project. Her keen eye and sharp pen have made me look like a much better writer than I am. My gratitude is also extended to John Sweet, Tilman Lewis and Gillian Watts.

I would be remiss if I didn't thank Jackie Kaiser, president of Westwood Creative Artists, my agent extraordinaire. She not only made the book happen quickly but handled my sometimes neurotic concerns (like "Do we need a clause in the contract covering what happens if I get Covid and die?") with aplomb.

I need to thank my colleagues at the *Globe and Mail*. The paper has a fabulous Covid-19 team that has been going full bore since January 2020. As a columnist, my work is often solitary and it's been an inspiration to be part of a group that has been so dogged and creative in covering this once-in-a-century pandemic. The paper's coverage of the crisis in LTC, in particular, has been stellar, and I've been lucky to take inspiration from it. If that were not enough, editors and reporters have been incredibly supportive of each other. That solidarity and camaraderie in a workplace is priceless.

At the risk of sounding immodest, I will say that there is much wisdom in this book. But it all comes from family caregivers, care providers and researchers who are featured. Like all of us, they were challenged and often overwhelmed by the pandemic, but still gave selflessly of their time.

One of the great privileges of being a journalist is being allowed into people's lives, often when they are under extreme duress. Some of the caregivers and workers I interviewed were stressed and sleepless, having been locked out of care homes because of the pandemic, or fearing for their lives; others were grieving a parent or spouse who had just died. Yet they shared intimacies, emotions and insights, in the hope that it would help spark reform and ensure others will not feel neglected and suffer as they and their loved ones have. That dedication and strength is awe-inspiring.

I can only hope that I have done their stories justice. And, most of all, my fervent wish is that those with the power to make the necessary changes to eldercare are listening and, at long last, willing to act.

Sources

Introduction

Eric Andrew-Gee and Laura Stone, "Understaffing turned seniors' homes into COVID-19 danger zones, health workers say. What can be done to fix that?" *Globe and Mail,* August 10, 2020.

André Picard, "Ineptitude killed 32 seniors. Only an orgy of inaction has followed," *Globe and Mail,* January 20, 2015.

Emma McIntosh, "Killer nurse Elizabeth Wettlaufer sentenced to life in prison," *Toronto Star,* June 26, 2017.

André Picard, "The long-term care system failed to prevent eight murders. The Wettlaufer inquiry failed by not holding anyone accountable," *Globe and Mail,* July 31, 2019.

Les Perreaux, "Snowstorm death of Duceppe's mother sparks Quebec coroner investigation," *Globe and Mail,* January 21, 2019.

André Picard, "When disaster strikes, you can count on politicians to call in the bureaucrats," *Globe and Mail,* January 30, 2014.

"Reimagining Long-Term Care," *Lancet* 396, no. 10259 (2020): P1307.

Chapter 1

André Picard, "Senior care facilities are especially vulnerable to COVID-19 outbreaks," *Globe and Mail*, March 8, 2020.

Aaron Derfel, "Public health, police find bodies, feces at Dorval seniors' residence: Sources," *Montreal Gazette*, April 11, 2020.

Paul Cherry, "Laval CHSLD hit hard by pandemic has recorded 100 deaths," *Montreal Gazette*, July 3, 2020.

Mike Hager and Andrea Woo, "How the coronavirus took North Vancouver's Lynn Valley Care," *Globe and Mail*, March 21, 2020.

Linda Gyulai, "Death toll reaches 51 at Résidence Herron; long coroner's probe expected," *Montreal Gazette*, May 21, 2020.

Kelly Grant, "Canada ranks among worst in OECD for long-term care deaths," *Globe and Mail*, June 25, 2020.

Carole Estabrooks, Colleen Flood, and Sharon Straus, "We must act now to prevent a second wave of long-term care deaths," *Globe and Mail*, June 10, 2020.

André Picard, "If you can get your relatives out of seniors' homes, try to do so as fast as you can," *Globe and Mail*, April 2, 2020.

André Picard, "Seniors' care shouldn't be a horror show, even after a pandemic," *Globe and Mail*, April 11, 2020.

"How Canada gave a pandemic the key to the country's nursing homes," editorial, *Globe and Mail*, April 14, 2020.

Moira Welsh, "'Everyone knew this could happen': The deadly spread of COVID-19 through Canada's seniors' homes," *Toronto Star*, April 15, 2020.

Jonathan Gatehouse, "Advocates wonder why long-term care COVID warnings were ignored," CBC News, April 14, 2020.

Tu Thanh Ha, "How Quebec's long-term care homes became hotbeds for the COVID-19 pandemic," *Globe and Mail*, May 7, 2020.

Tu Thanh Ha, Les Perreaux, and Eric Andrew-Gee, "Coroner, health authorities and police launch investigations into Montreal nursing home after 31 seniors die," *Globe and Mail*, April 12, 2020.

Kathleen Harris and Ashley Burke, "The long-term care crisis: How B.C. controlled COVID-19 while Ontario, Quebec face disaster," CBC News, May 28, 2020.

Kelly Grant and Jill Mahoney, "A postmortem for Pinecrest: How systemic flaws led to tragedy at a Bobcaygeon nursing home," *Globe and Mail*, May 1, 2020.

Dan Bilefsky, "31 deaths: Toll at Quebec nursing home in pandemic reflects global phenomenon," *New York Times*, April 16, 2020.

Karen Howlett, Jill Mahoney, and Laura Stone, "Infestations, sedation and neglect: Military report details 'horrific' living conditions in seniors' homes," *Globe and Mail*, May 26, 2020.

Tu Thanh Ha, "Inspection reports reveal critical gaps inside Quebec nursing homes ravaged by COVID-19," *Globe and Mail*, May 26, 2020.

André Picard, "If Doug Ford wants long-term care reform, he should be bold and decisive and just do it," *Globe and Mail*, May 26, 2020.

Chapter 2

Norma Rudy, *For Such a Time as This: L. Earl Ludlow and a History of Homes for the Aged in Ontario 1837–1961* (Ontario Association of Homes for the Aged, 1987).

Taylor Alexander, "The History and Evolution of Long-Term Care in Canada," in *Continuing the Care: The Issues and Challenges for Long-Term Care*, ed. Eleanor Sawyer (Ottawa: CHA Press, 2002), pp. 1–53.

Pat Armstrong et al., *They Deserve Better: The Long-Term Care Experience in Canada and Scandinavia* (Ottawa: Canadian Centre for Policy Alternatives, 2009).

Amy Twomey, "The Marginalization of Long-Term Care in Canadian Federal Policy Making," PhD candidate in Canadian Studies, Trent University, 2010.

Canadian Forces Advisory Council, *The Origins and Evolution of Veterans Benefits in Canada 1914–2004* (Ottawa: Veterans Affairs Canada, 2004).

Albert Banerjee, *An Overview of Long-Term Care in Canada and Selected Provinces and Territories: Women and Health Care Reform* (October 2007).

Chapter 3

Working Group on Long-Term Care, *Restoring Trust: COVID-19 and the Future of Long-Term Care* (Ottawa: Royal Society of Canada, 2020).

Pat Armstrong, Hugh Armstrong, Jacqueline Choiniere, Ruth Lowndes, and James Struthers, *Re-imagining Long-Term Residential Care in the Covid-19 Crisis* (Toronto: April 2020).

C.A. Estabrooks, J.E. Squires, H.L. Carleton, G.G. Cummings, and P.G. Norton, "Who Is Looking After Mom and Dad? Unrelegulated Workers in Canadian Long-Term Care Homes," *Canadian Journal on Aging* 34, no. 1 (2015): 47–59.

Dr. Samir Sinha, *Living Longer, Living Well*, report submitted to the Minister of Health and Long-Term Care and the Minister Responsible for Seniors on recommendations to inform a seniors' strategy in Ontario, December 12, 2013.

National Institute on Ageing, *Canada Is Not Keeping Pace with the Home and Community, and Nursing Home Care Needs of Its Rapidly Ageing Population* (Toronto: National Institute on Ageing, 2019).

Dr. Samir Sinha et al., *Enabling the Future Provision of Long-Term Care in Canada* (Toronto: National Institute on Ageing, 2019).

Moira Welsh, "Should long-term care homes be 'old-person storage' or places to live?" *Toronto Star*, August 17, 2020.

Kathy Tomlinson and Grant Robertson, "It took a pandemic: Why systemic deficiencies in long-term care facilities pose such a danger to seniors," *Globe and Mail*, April 27, 2020.

Richard Mollot, "Nursing homes were a disaster waiting to happen," *New York Times*, April 28, 2020.

Moira Welsh, "Covid-19 has exposed problems in long-term care: Will the response fix it?" *Toronto Star*, April 29, 2020.

"Canada's long-term care home system 'designed to produce mediocrity', says health policy expert," *Cross-Country Checkup*, CBC Radio, May 31, 2020.

Martin Regg Cohn, "When it comes to long-term care, what matters more than ownership is accountability and responsibility," *Toronto Star*, May 11, 2020.

Thomas Gerbet, "Plus d'inspecteurs pour veiller au bien-être des animaux qu'à celui des aînés," Radio-Canada Info, June 23, 2020.

Crisis Point: Addressing the Needs of Seniors Living in Long-Term Care (Canadian Association for Long-Term Care, 2020).

Pat Armstrong et al., *Models for Long-Term Residential Care: A Summary of the Consultants' Report to Long-Term Care Homes and Services, City of Toronto*, April 15, 2019.

Chapter 4

Madhuri Reddy, Nathan Stall, and Paula Rochon, "How coronavirus could forever change home health care, leaving vulnerable older adults without care and overburdening caregivers," *Policy Options*, May 18, 2020.

Lauren Vogel, "The home care conversation we're not having," CMAJ, June 26, 2017, 189 (25) E875–E876.

Brian Platt, "As COVID-19 ravages nursing homes, researcher warns that home-care patients can't be forgotten," *National Post*, April 17, 2020.

David Fisman, MD, MPH, et al., *Failing Our Most Vulnerable: COVID-19 and Long-Term Care Facilities in Ontario* (Ottawa: Canadian Institutes of Health Research, 2020).

John Hirdes et al., "Derivation and Validation of the Personal Support Algorithm: An Evidence-Based Framework to Inform Allocation of Personal Support Services in Home and Community Care," *BMC Health Services Research* 17 (2017): 775.

André Picard, "In the stay-at-home era, why have we so sorely neglected home care?" *Globe and Mail*, June 15, 2020.

Carly Weeks, "Why the future of health care may depend on tearing down the hospital," *Globe and Mail*, February 21, 2014.

Chapter 5

Prevalence and Monetary Costs of Dementia in Canada (Toronto: Alzheimer Society of Canada, 2016).

Esther Landhuis, "Is Dementia Risk Falling?" *Scientific American*, January 25, 2016.

A Dementia Strategy for Canada: Together We Aspire (Ottawa: Public Health Agency of Canada, 2019).

Paula Rochon and Jaimie Roebuck, "Is Canada's dementia strategy set up to fail?" *Globe and Mail*, July 22, 2019.

Parul Sehgal, "Dementia patients aren't in their 'perfect mind.' Then again, who is?" *New York Times*, April 21, 2020.

Larry W. Chambers, Christina Bancej, and Ian McDowell, eds., *Prevalence and Monetary Cost of Dementia in Canada* (Toronto: Alzheimer Society of Canada, 2016).

Gill Livingston et al., "Dementia Prevention, Intervention, and Care: 2020 Report of the Lancet Commission," *Lancet*, July 30, 2020.

Lynn Casteel Harper, *On Vanishing: Mortality, Dementia, and What It Means to Disappear* (New York: Catapult, 2020).

Chapter 6

Minister's Expert Advisory Panel on Long Term Care (Nova Scotia), Janice Keefe, chair, December 21, 2018.

Carole Estabrooks and Janice Keefe, "The human face of care aides in Canada," *Vancouver Province*, April 25, 2020.

Shaina Luck, "Long-term care workers were already overloaded. Then the pandemic came," CBC News, June 15, 2020.

Anne Jarvis, "The front-line care workers you don't hear about," *Windsor Star*, April 16, 2020.

Andrew Pinto, Pinky Hapsari, and Debra Slater, "Lack of protection for personal support workers emblematic of their treatment in the system," *Toronto Star*, April 14, 2020.

Terrie Laplante-Beauchamp, "Three days of death and disorder: A Montreal orderly's diary from a nursing home's coronavirus outbreak," *Globe and Mail*, April 15, 2020.

Michelle Lalonde, "Pay hikes alone won't end shortage of personal care workers: Experts," *Montreal Gazette*, April 21, 2020.

Marcus Gee, "Let's value our personal support workers," *Globe and Mail*, April 24, 2020.

Nicolas Keung and Jason Miller, "Until COVID-19 hit, PSWs went virtually unnoticed," *Toronto Star*, May 1, 2020.

Johanna Wolfert and Brian Dijkema, *Structural Challenges to Personal Support Worker Funding* (Hamilton, ON: Cardus, 2020).

Ian DaSilva, *The Personal Support Worker in Ontario 2001–2017: An Occupation in Crisis* (Cambridge, ON: Ontario Personal Support Workers Association, 2019).

Cheryl Chan and Tara Carman, "9 out of 10 seniors facilities in B.C. don't meet staffing guidelines," *Vancouver Sun*, January 26, 2017.

Alison Motluk, "Self-Regulation in Health Care Professions Comes under Scrutiny," *Canadian Medical Association Journal*, July 30, 2019.

Chapter 7

Nathan Stall, "We should care more about caregivers," CMAJ, March 4, 2019, 191 (9) E245–E246, doi.org/10.1503/cmaj.190204.

André Picard, "Unpaid caregivers do a lot of heavy lifting—and they deserve more support," *Globe and Mail*, November 20, 2018.

Caregivers in Distress: A Growing Problem (Victoria: Office of the Seniors Advocate, 2017).

Caregivers in Canada, 2018, Statistics Canada, January 8, 2020.

Benjamin Tal, "Who will care for Canada's caregivers?" *Globe and Mail*, February 25, 2019.

Zosia Bielski, "With a looming aging crisis, who is helping the caregivers?" *Globe and Mail*, April 13, 2019.

Chapter 8

Amit Arya, "Palliative care has been lacking for decades in long-term care," *Policy Options*, July 16, 2020.

Access to Palliative Care in Canada (Ottawa: Canadian Institute for Health Information, 2018).

Marilyn A. Mendoza, "What Is a Good Death? How to Die Well," *Psychology Today*, March 14, 2020.

André Picard, "There are a lot better places to die than Canada," *Globe and Mail*, July 21, 2010.

Kelly Grant, "Medically assisted death allows couple married almost 73 years to die together," *Globe and Mail*, April 1, 2018.

Darren Cargill, "Palliative care needs better PR," *Healthy Debate*, August 26, 2020.

Darren Cargill, "Palliative care training 'woefully inadequate' in meeting need," *Healthy Debate*, July 2, 2020.

Janice Legere, "Virus vs. visitors: Why long-term care needs a palliative approach," *Healthy Debate*, August 6, 2020.

Chapter 9

Ian MacAlpine, "Oasis program for seniors expanding to other Ontario communities," *Kingston Whig-Standard*, November 23, 2018.

Diarmaid Ward, "Jane Jacobs and Le Corbusier would agree on one thing: we need more social housing," *CityMetric*, September 23, 2019.

Catherine Donnelly, Paul Nguyen, Simone Parniak, and Vincent DePaul, "Beyond long-term care: The benefits of seniors' communities that evolve on their own," *Conversation Canada*, September 8, 2020.

Paul J. Masotti, Robert Fick, Ana Johnson-Masott, and Stuart MacLeod, "Healthy Naturally Occurring Retirement Communities: A Low-Cost Approach to Facilitating Healthy Aging," *American Journal of Public Health* 96, no. 7 (2006): 1164–70.

Chief Public Health Officer of Canada, *Health Status of Canadians 2016* (Ottawa: Public Health Agency of Canada, 2016).

Chapter 10

Magnus Heunicke, Stephanie Lose, and Jete Kive, *A Dignified Elderly Care in Denmark* (Odense, Denmark: Healthcare Denmark, 2019).

International Health Care System Profiles (New York: Commonwealth Fund, 2019).

John Muscedere et al., "Frailty and Ageing: Canadian Challenges and Lessons Learned in Denmark," *Longwoods Healthcare Quarterly*, Spring 2018.

André Picard, "Some harsh lessons on the failings of eldercare from Down Under," *Globe and Mail*, November 12, 2019.

Ilango Ponnuswami and Rangasamy Rajasekaran, "Long-Term Care of Older Persons in India: Learning to Deal with Challenges," *International Journal on Ageing in Developing Countries* 2, no. 1 (2017): 59–71.

Blanche Le Bihan and Claude Martin, "French Social and Long Term Care System," *Global Social Security Review* 7 (Winter 2018): 5–15.

Judy Steed, "Elderly thrive in Denmark," *Toronto Star*, November 9, 2008.

Chapter 11

Sandra Martin, "How one hospital is dealing with Canada's aging population," *Globe and Mail*, January 24, 2014.

Sandra Martin, "Veterans at Sunnybrook show us how to age gracefully," *Globe and Mail*, December 5, 2013.

Nadine Yousif, "Sunnybrook hospital celebrates 70 years of veterans' care," *Globe and Mail*, June 11, 2018.

Colin Perkel, "Sunnybrook Veterans Centre under federal audit following accusations of neglect," *Globe and Mail*, December 21, 2012.

Veterans Affairs Canada, Veterans Independence Program, January 11, 2019.

Veterans Health Care Regulations (Ottawa: Minister of Justice, 2019).

Index

MAID (medical assistance in
dying), 129, 130–31
Major, Bill, 121–22
Major, Marilyn, 121–22
Marquez, Josephine, 93–97
Marshall, Audrey, 157–58
Marshall, Jack, 156–58
Martin, Paul, 63–64
Masterson, Deiren, 114, 115–17, 118
Masterson, Maureen, 114–15
Masterson, Paul, 114, 115, 116–17
McCann, Danielle, 17
McVey, Lynne, 13
Mialkowski, C.J.J., 20–21
mini-strokes (TIAs), 78
Montreal Gazette, 13, 16, 17
Mount, Balfour, 127–28
Mount Sinai Hospital (Toronto), 109
Mule, Loredana, 13–14

National Advisory Committee on
SARS, 11–12
*National Evaluation of the
Cost-Effectiveness of Home
Care* (Hollander and
Chappell), 74
Naylor, David, 11–12
Netherlands, 153
New Brunswick, 101
Newfoundland and Labrador, 103
Nicin, Michael, 173
Noël, André, 40
NORCs (naturally occurring
retirement communities),
138–40
Norway, 35, 153
Nova Scotia, 97, 110
nurses, 122, 177
and eldercare, 98, 159–60, 164–65
nursing homes, 49, 168–69. *See also*
long-term-care homes
in Denmark, 146, 147–48

Oasis Senior Supportive Living
(Kingston, ON), 138–39
old age security, 112
Omapas, Jovencio, 110–11, 112
Ontario, 11. *See also* Ontario
legislation; Toronto
Covid-19 care-home deaths,
22–24, 27
health care spending, 66
health profession regulation,
102–3
home care in, 66, 67
Local Health Integration
Networks (LHINs), 54
long-term care in, 28–33, 50,
52–54, 80–81, 100, 170
personal care workers in, 95–96
Ontario legislation
Homes for the Aged Act, 31–32
Long-Term Care Act, 100
Nursing Home Act (1966), 32–33

pain management, 123–24
palliative care, 120–30
access to, 120, 126, 128, 129
elements of, 123, 124–25, 129
at home, 120
in hospice, 127–28
in hospitals, 121, 124, 126
improving, 170–71
long-term care and, 120, 126
problems with, 122–24
Palmer, Frank and Irene, 61, 67–70
pandemics, 10, 12, 25–26. *See also
specific diseases*
personal care workers, 92–104. *See
also* nurses; PSWs; *specific
work contexts*
in British Columbia, 95–96, 97,
103
client needs, 93–94
Covid-19 and, 26, 95, 98, 121

ANDRÉ PICARD is a health reporter and columnist for the *Globe and Mail*, where he has been a staff writer since 1987. He is also the author of five bestselling books. André is an eight-time nominee for the National Newspaper Awards, Canada's top journalism prize, and past winner of a prestigious Michener Award for Meritorious Public Service Journalism. He was named Canada's first "Public Health Hero" by the Canadian Public Health Association, and a "Champion of Mental Health" by the Canadian Alliance on Mental Illness and Mental Health, and received the Queen Elizabeth II Diamond Jubilee Medal for his dedication to improving health care. André is a graduate of the University of Ottawa and Carleton University, and has received honorary doctorates from six universities, including UBC and the University of Toronto.